2·25·74

KEEP TRYING

KEEP TRYING

a practical book
for the handicapped
by a polio victim

JOSEPH LAURANCE MARX

HARPER & ROW, PUBLISHERS

New York, Evanston, San Francisco, London

FIRST EDITION

Designed by Gwendolyn O. England

Library of Congress Cataloging in Publication Data

Marx, Joseph Laurance.
  Keep trying; a practical book for the handicapped.
  Bibliography: p. 197
  1. Poliomyelitis—Personal narratives. I. Title.
RC180.2.M33   362.4'3'0924 [B]   73–4107
ISBN 0–06–012827–5

1799183

For Dorothy

Contents

Acknowledgments

Thanks . . .

So many people and organizations have been helpful by giving me information and some of their precious time that I cannot possibly thank them all.

I am not listing many medical people who have worked on me in the past, some of whom are mentioned in the text and to whom I am grateful for the efforts that enabled me to become ambulatory and stay alive. I wish to thank in particular a few people who were especially helpful in giving me information and material. These would include Dr. Sam Sverdlik, Dr. Leon Greenspan, and Dr. Thomas A. Doyle, Miss Henrietta Buckmaster, Mrs. Jerome Flexner, and a number of people connected with the Veterans Administration in New York and Washington, with Bellevue and the New York University Hospital, with Alcoholics Anonymous, the Council on Alcoholism, Abilities, Inc., and my sister, Jeanne, who read a draft of this book and prodded my memory on some aspects.

All my thanks to these, and many others.

J. L. M.

Preface

It was not my idea to write this book. I've been a writer for a number of years, but writing a book of this type had not occurred to me. It was suggested, and my immediate reaction was no. It's not that I'm modest, but I felt that doing a book of this type would make it appear that I thought I was important enough to be worth writing about. After some time, I changed my mind, not because I thought I was any more important, but because I realized I had strong feelings and opinions on some of the problems with which a handicapped person has to cope.

I had polio about sixty years ago, when I was between three and four years old. It struck very suddenly, as is characteristic, and left me with one badly twisted leg and foot, and another that was fairly straight but thin, as it has almost no muscles. Since then, I have led what seems to have been an active life. I've been married twice, have helped bring up four daughters, all of whom are married now with children of their own. I learned how to drive a car when that was more difficult to do with or without two good legs, and, later, to fly a plane.

I have traveled extensively, by plane, train, or automobile, in all of the contiguous United States, Latin America, the Caribbean, and Western Europe. I have been the editor of a newspaper feature syndicate and of several magazines, worked for the government, run a large news room, written sports, reviewed plays, covered night clubs and restaurants and national and international affairs, written short stories and articles for many national magazines, and had several books published.

What I'm trying to say is that I have led quite an active "normal" life professionally and socially, and look forward to doing so for some time to come. I'm on good terms with a large number of people, famous, infamous, or unknown outside their own circles. I'm on a couple of committees at my college (Columbia) and am president of my alumni class. In other words, I get around.

I changed my mind and decided to write this book because I thought that, by going back into my experiences and those of others I've known, I might be able to offer some thoughts and ideas and methods that could be useful to the handicapped, and even more so to those who are apt to cause the handicapped most of their troubles—their friends, relatives, and co-workers.

The use of the word "he" throughout is impersonal and genderless. It is used the way the word "man" is or was, short for mankind. To say "he or she" every time is clumsy and "one" is often too impersonal. I will say "he" when "he" means "someone."

I realized when working on this that my outlook may sound like that of a Pollyanna or at times somewhat mystical, but I am firmly convinced that the most important factor for a physically handicapped person is not what he is able to do but his attitude. And that what he is able to do is more dependent on his attitude than on his physical abilities. That his own attitude determines how other people regard him. And that, within certain well-defined limits, if a handicapped person wants badly enough to do something, he'll work out a way to do it.

It's hard to write a book like this without seeming to be saying, "Look at me—see what I have done." If it sounds like that at times, it is not out of pride but out of a desire to show others a way they can do certain things.

In a way, I feel like a phony writing a book about the handicapped, because I have met so many people who have had to overcome problems much worse than mine. This is not a false disclaimer—it's just that I have grown so accustomed to what I can and cannot do that I don't think about it, and someone with a different handicap might think what I do is as remarkable as I consider his accomplishments. The main thing I have done, I think, is to have survived a number of what might have been traumatic experiences with comparatively little distortion of my psyche. Starting with an abnormal situation, I have led a full and gratifying life. Generally speaking, I have enjoyed myself, I enjoy myself now, and I look forward to tomorrow, next week, next year, and the rest of my life.

I say I have been lucky, and I will say it repeatedly because I feel it. I was and am lucky in my family, my friends, and my situation in general.

J.L.M.

New York City
December 1973

CHAPTER ONE

In the Beginning

This story began in 1913, when I was about three and one-half years old and came down with poliomyelitis, which was then called infantile paralysis. My disease was not correctly diagnosed until many months later, which was unimportant, as at that time there was no useful early treatment. Today, the ailment has almost disappeared in the United States because of the Salk and Sabin immunizing sera.

I remember, or think I remember, many of the things I write about, although it is not easy to be sure whether what one considers a memory is not actually something one heard about. I can remember certain things before I contracted polio, because there was a sharp break in my activities at that time. My grandfather, for instance, coming by on his horse and asking me to turn a somersault and then a "peppersault" (his word for a backward somersault) before he'd pick me up and hold me in his saddle for a short ride. I can remember the day I came down with the disease. I had been taken out for a ride in the country, with some of my family, in a White Steamer (not a Stanley Steamer). When we arrived home, I was sick and in pain, and had to be lifted out of the car and carried into the house and put to bed.

I had had diphtheria some time before, and at first it was thought I was having a delayed relapse. It rapidly got worse. I might add that I am not going solely by my memory. My mother has kept a brief daily diary from the time she was a teen-ager and still does today, in her upper eighties. When I knew I was going to write this, I borrowed her diaries and excerpted some pertinent items from them. The entries follow, with the dates. The year was 1913.

JUNE 11   Joseph has bad throat.

JUNE 14   Right after lunch, Dick calls for O [my father], the two kiddies and me and we go to the country. Olive Street Road, White Horse Creek Road, Manchester Road home.

JUNE 17   Joseph has all the symptoms of diphtheria. JC to Grandma's for a while. [JC was my older sister, Jeanne.]

JUNE 18   Nurse Joseph.

JUNE 19   Nurse Joseph. Not diphtheria but diphtheroid nose. [A small item in different-colored ink underneath says: "Months later. Know now it was infantile paralysis."]

JUNE 20   Just stay home and nurse Joseph.

JUNE 21   Joseph's legs go back on him. Infection affected kidneys which affect legs. Can't walk.

JUNE 22   Bad day with Joseph. Jeanne came home for dinner but went back to grandmother's.

JUNE 23   Nurse Joseph.

JUNE 24   Joseph in bad shape. Can't even sit up or move legs. Sweeney in the afternoon. [That was Miss Sweeney, a trained nurse who came home from the hospital with

my sister first, then with me, and years later with my
brother when he was born. I remember her as a capable, warmhearted woman. She died years ago.]

JUNE 25 Joseph moves only arms.

JUNE 26 Didn't sleep five minutes as nursing high fever.

This entry is repeated until:

JULY 1 Joseph better.

Then, at times: "Joseph better" or "has bad day.
. . ."

JULY 26 Dad calls for Jeanne and me. Take ride. Then take
Joseph for first auto ride.

DEC. 11 Busy with Joseph all day. He walks in street today with
braces and crutches, first time without being held.

I am using my mother's diaries for two reasons: as a mne-
monic aid, and to show the speed with which the disease
spread once it got started. On June 11, I had a bad throat,
which evidently improved because on June 14 I was able to
go for a ride in the country. Three days after that, I seemed
to have all the symptoms of diphtheria. Four days later, I
couldn't walk. Ten days after the ride in the country, I
couldn't even sit up. Six months after that, I walked on the
street with braces and crutches.

In those six months, my life had changed completely. I had
moved from one world to another. I have spent a portion of
my years since working my way back to that other, more
usual world.

There is no question about it, the world of the handicapped
is a different world. The billions of humans living on this
planet are divided and united by many factors. We are white,
black, yellow, red, brown, or shades in between. To a certain
extent, we all live in different and separate worlds, with
subdivisions for poor or rich, male or female, for people of
different religions, customs, beliefs, and ways of living, speak-

ing languages that are different but understandable (Cockney-Yorkshire, Yankee-Dixie) or that are similar but not understandable (Spanish-Portuguese).

With all the divisions there are, with all the different worlds separating and unifying people, there are few so sharply defined and so unyielding in their perimeters as the area separating the physically handicapped from the physically normal. I have lived as a bridge between these worlds in a manner satisfactory to me. While doing this, I have learned some things about these two worlds, and I think I might be able to make life easier and more understandable for some inhabitants of both.

I was lucky. Not because I was suddenly moved from one world to another, but in other ways. First, because I lived. Second, because of my parents. Maybe they weren't lucky, but I was, because they were intelligent and not poor. They were exceptionally thoughtful, aware people whose treatment of my problems was several decades ahead of what might have been expected. And they were secure enough in their finances so they could do for me what they wanted to do. That was in a day when medical financing was almost totally private or charitable, with noticeable differences in attitudes and quality.

What kind of material did they have to work with? They had what had been a bright and active little boy. I'm not overly modest: I'm no genius, but I was never considered stupid. At the time I was hit by polio, I was a medium-sized, wiry kid. Suddenly, I was immobile. Polio strikes in its own fashion, and if it doesn't kill, its worst damage comes in the aftereffects. I was left with a normally shaped but generally muscleless left leg, and a right leg that had a few working muscles but had been twisted out of shape, almost like a clubfoot. So my left side was almost ignored while the doctors concentrated on doing what they could to make my right leg usable.

From that point on, my education changed. The early years of most people are spent in learning to live with the world. From birth, one is adjusting or not adjusting to the environment into which one has been thrust. This includes learning acceptable ways of behavior—eating, drinking, expressing one's thoughts, wishes, and needs. A natural part of this is learning to walk and run and play with one's peers. My education had to include these things and some others. I spent a large amount of time in bed, at home or in hospitals. I had to learn to walk, not once but several times. I had to learn how to be alone a good deal of the time, and I had to learn how to live with pain.

It has been said that suffering ennobles. I don't think it does. It may seem to ennoble some who have suffered, but we have no way of knowing how these same people would have turned out if they had been spared agony. There is little doubt in my mind that suffering can twist, warp, and embitter. I remember running across a character in a book who had been maimed by some misfortune. He spent his time carving or whittling tiny humanlike figures and, after finishing them, crumbling them in his hand, saying or thinking, "I am God." I remember thinking what an odd idea of God he must have.

The character-building, ennobling aspect of suffering has always seemed to me to be an expression by the nonsufferer of "Thank God, he's got it, not I." By seeming to find a virtue in suffering—someone else's suffering, of course—the nonsufferer can avoid the necessity of thinking about it or empathizing with it. It is well known to most people that others do not feel the way we do—the other man has a capacity to withstand pain that we do not have, particularly if he is of a different nationality, color, or religion. The fabled "sweet uses of adversity" are particularly beneficial, like poverty, for other people.

As with everything else in our changing world, the types of handicap that afflict mankind have changed over the centuries, and in this, too, the rate of change has been fastest in the past half-century. Polio, which had been a major crippler, has almost disappeared in the United States, the way small-pox has, or tuberculosis, or pellegra. As diseases have changed, the types of handicapped have changed. And be-cause the word "handicap" is a general one, the statistics on the subject are vague and unreliable.

At one time, without accurate statistics, it was estimated that the bulk of the physically handicapped got into that category because of disease or birth injury. Today, leaving out those who are incapacitated because of emotional prob-lems, the greatest crippler is accidents. And that goes not only for the United States but for the world. According to a United Nations report, there are close to three hundred mil-lion physically handicapped people in the world—almost one person out of every ten. In the United States and Western Europe, more than half of the injuries are the result of au-tomobile accidents, with another third coming from indus-trial and work accidents. Back in the "good old days" when the death-and-injury rate was not driven up by automobiles, the number of deaths and injuries caused by the then chief employer, agriculture, was much higher than it is now, in totals as well as in the percentage of people engaged in it. One accident factor that seems to have remained fairly con-stant is the percentage of disabling or disfiguring accidents that occur in the home.

One of the reasons statistics on this subject are unreliable is that handicaps are apt to be lumped together. A person with a mild handicap who can function pretty well but not perfectly is likely to be in the same classification as a person with a severe brain or nerve injury who can do next to nothing for himself. About the only "ratings" of the handicapped are a matter of money—the percentage of disability as shown by insurance figures or by the Veterans Administration figures for service-connected disabilities. Or in matters of sight, which can be measured on a scale of 0–100 percent.

Otherwise, disabilities and handicaps are difficult to measure, because it is impossible to evaluate them objectively. The amount of impairment caused by a specific disability depends on the individual, his vocation, his personality, his determination. A lawyer who is totally deaf, for instance, may be a brilliant legalist who turns out convincing briefs, but would be at a great disadvantage as a trial attorney. Should he be considered to be suffering from a major disability, a minor one, or none at all?

Most handicaps or disabilities are not easy to measure; how bad they are depends on how they are handled.

CHAPTER TWO

Know Thyself

I am writing for and about handicapped people—primarily those with motor-skeletal handicaps, those who have difficulty getting around, problems with their arms and legs—and for their friends, families, and acquaintances.

The subject of this book is the struggle for rehabilitation: to help those with a physical problem get back on their feet, whether that is done physically or metaphorically, to help them lead a happier, more normal, more useful life. The first move in this direction is contained in the two-word chapter heading. Sooner or later, everyone has to discover what he can do and, just as important, what he can't do. For a person with a handicap, this has to come sooner rather than later.

This seems so elementary it might look like a waste of time to mention it much less to stress it. It isn't. I put it first because I think it is of primary importance in building a life that is full of the usual number of satisfactions and frustrations. I don't like to use the word "normal" because it is loosely defined and used, but I can find no other word that says the same thing so succinctly. Because the first thing a handicapped person has to face is that in the eyes of the world he isn't normal.

The role of any individual in our complicated world is a complex one. The idea of growing up, reaching maturity, finding one's identity, is a matter of discovering one's capabilities, of adjusting one's aspirations within tolerable limits of effectiveness. Some people discover this at an early age, some mature late, some never. That doesn't mean aspirations must be cut down to a minimum, it just means that they should not be set so high that life is going to be a constant disappointment. This is true all the way through the life of a handicapped person, possibly to a greater degree than it is true of other people. There has to be hope and there has to be a delicate adjustment between hope, dreams, and reality. The handicapped, if their troubles come to them young, have to make this adjustment earlier than others.

Most people have to adjust their dreams to reality. This is often called growing up, reaching maturity, or being sensible. Most boys like to daydream of being a Mickey Mantle or Wilt Chamberlain or an airline pilot, just as in an earlier day they dreamed of being a cowboy or railroad engineer or steamboat pilot, realizing they probably never would be; the handicapped boy has the same dreams, but he *knows* at an earlier age that he is not going to lead a glamorous life if it entails exceptional physical skills.

The physically handicapped child has to live even more in his imagination than most children. This is fine as a safety valve, as a method of escaping a reality that otherwise might seem to be unbearable—as long as the dreamer realizes he is dreaming, and why. If that isn't the case, he can slip over the line into total unreality. Sometimes this happens because stupid or unknowing people try to be helpful.

I can recall two children who received, for different problems, totally different kinds of adult help, one kind almost ruinous, one very useful. They were both girls. One had had a crippling ailment. A series of complications developed so that she had to have an amputation. At the time, she was a good young Catholic, in a good old Catholic hospital. She was naturally upset when she heard the news. The night before her operation was scheduled, one of the older Sisters came to talk to her. This well-meaning lady told the little girl that she would be all right—she was so young, prayers would be said for her, and with her youth and the prayers, a new limb would probably grow in as a replacement.

I met this little girl perhaps twenty years later. I had noticed her, after seeing her several times at a place we were both going for treatment, because she seemed to be particularly withdrawn and bitter. In due time, without my asking, the story came out. "I was eight at the time and old enough to know better," she said. "I don't think I really believed it then, but it was a Sister telling me, and I wanted so badly to believe it that I did." She explained that, no matter how she tried afterward, she never regained her pristine faith or recovered completely from her disillusionment.

The other case was much simpler. A little girl was born with six toes. For reasons medically sound at the time, the extra digit was not removed. Her mother worried, as the child grew older, that when she started to go to school, the extra toe might cause problems if it were noticed and commented on. So she told the little girl that it was a lucky sign, like the extra leaf in a four-leaf clover. At the time when the girl first started undressing in school for naps or swimming, instead of being shy about it she was always taking off one shoe and sock and explaining, "See? I'm lucky. I've got an extra toe."

There's a major difference between having one toe too many and one limb too few, but the differentiation that made the difference was more one of attitude than one of a physical plus or minus. Of course, you can't tell a little girl who has lost or is about to lose her lower leg that she is lucky. But you shouldn't be able to tell her she will grow a new one. It is nice to tell a distressed and worried child something that will cheer her up and make her feel better. But it should never be anything that will prove to be false.

Common sense would tell you that, but I knew, too, from personal experience when I was quite young. My attack of polio had left me in poor shape. I couldn't move about much, and had to be helped even to sit up. After I was able to do that alone, my mobility was limited to ways I could move myself, using my arms and hands. We lived in St. Louis in a fairly large house in a nice residential neighborhood. I spent much of my time in bed or going to doctors or getting fitted for orthopedic appliances. Eventually, wearing special shoes and braces, I was able to walk after a fashion, using crutches. The braces fitted into places built for them at the heels of the shoes, and locked at the hip and knee so that I could put my weight on either leg without having the joint buckle. With these, and with crutches and caution, I could move about a bit, although my speed resembled a glacier's rather than that of a snail.

Nevertheless, every fair morning, I went out for a walk with my mother. An innovative woman, she devised a pair of crutches and had them built with extensions above the shoulder pieces so that, walking behind me, she could help me move the crutches, or even move them for me. Our house was in the middle of the block, and a very long walk, in time consumed, would be to the corner and back. I did not then have the control of my body I had later.

Thinking about those early walks, I remember that a dozen years later, when I was in college, I had a crutch race with a classmate, an aspiring pole-vaulter who had committed the unpardonable sin for a vaulter—he'd broken an ankle in a bad landing. I'd given him a few tips about walking on crutches when he'd had to start using them, so after he'd been doing it for a few weeks, he challenged me to a race. It was held on a cinder track in front of the dorms, fairly late at night, before what might be called a mixed audience— partly invited and partly there by accident. The fact that I beat him wasn't important—I should have, I was more ex- perienced. But the memory of that race makes me realize how far I'd come since the time when a one-block walk took between one and two hours. Incidentally, although he was a fine athlete, I was never able to teach him my little trick of walking on crutches without letting my feet touch the ground, a stunt I could keep up on level but not slippery terrain for a couple of hundred feet, with luck. He was never able to make more than ten or twelve feet that way, but he was suffering from a handicap—he had started too late in life.

Quite early in my recovery, I went to the hospital in St. Louis for an operation. It sticks out in my mind for two reasons: one was that the recovery period was very painful, the other was that I had somehow believed that it was going to accomplish miracles. The operation had to do with slitting a tendon or two, to help straighten my foot and leg, and recovery was long and tedious. Somehow I'd been led to think that I was going to be able to walk again after that operation. My parents had never said so, but that was the impression I had gained. Through the period of recuperation, I was buoyed up by the idea of running and playing like other boys. That wasn't very realistic of me, but I very much wanted to run and play. At the age of six, what else is important?

My mother's diary does not go into any detail about the operation. It mentions taking me to the hospital one evening, and the next day says, "J. operated this morning . . . stretch tendons and place bones." For the next few days, it says, I was miserable, and then better, and then a few weeks later was taken home from the hospital and continued being either miserable or uncomfortable. Almost exactly a month after the operation, a single entry reports that my cast was removed and another put on. Three weeks after that, the new cast was removed, and a few days later the entry shows that I went to be fitted for a new brace and some shoes. By that time, I knew that I was not going to be able to walk much better than I had before the operation. I never spoke about my disappointment, nor did anyone, as I remember. The orthopedic surgeon gravely said, "It's an improvement, not as much as I had hoped."

Many years and many operations later, I realized that the operation just mentioned, while not a success according to my expectations, was not a failure. It was just the first of a long series of steps that had to be taken to rebuild my legs. What was wrong was only that I took optimistic forecasts, which were not meant for me, to be a true telling of the way it would be. For a number of reasons, I did not react like the little girl who had an amputation. The only effect it has had on me, I think, was to build up an ingrained skepticism, which is not a bad thing for a newsman and a writer to have. It helped give me an attitude I can only describe as "Check everything." I listen, without hostility and with interest, and believe very little of what anyone says until I can check it out.

I'm willing to listen, to be amused, entertained, or educated by what other people say, but I accept only a certain percentage of it as true.

Though I spent a large part of my childhood unable to move around very well or with any speed, I do not remember it as an unhappy period. I had a family—kind, intelligent parents, a slightly older sister and later a younger brother, loving grandparents, some cousins and assorted real and courtesy aunts and uncles. And friends. It wasn't a normal childhood because I didn't go to school very much, and didn't stay in any one school for any length of time. I had a series of teachers and tutors, and for some years a fine young woman as a governess.

Generally, I was in and out of a series of private schools. Although my parents believed in the public school system, it wasn't flexible enough to take in someone who would leave every six weeks or so to go see his doctor in Boston and might be out for long periods having operations. And there was always the question of where to put me: with little formal schooling, in what grade did I belong?

But that came later. Before that, I was in bed or at home alone, except for the family and help. One thing that did for me was get me into the habit of reading, a habit I've never tried to break. I was and am a compulsive reader, one of those people who will read every word on the back of a cereal box or in a week-old newspaper if nothing else is available. I didn't realize how much I had read until I got to college and discovered that most of the compulsory reading put before me was familiar material. I had missed certain aspects of formal education, things like penmanship and the multiplication tables. Today, my handwriting is terrible, my arithmetic fine, and my grammar a matter of ear rather than the rules, as I never had to parse sentences.

I'm sure my feelings about education were shaped by what happened to me. I'm all for it, but I think that in most cases what we get from it depends on what we bring to it. If we're fortunate enough to come from a family that is literate and interested, most of our educational battle is won. The people who work for an education, in my opinion, are those who come from families who do not speak well, who do not read as a matter of habit and enjoyment, who do not make any effort to keep up with current affairs that don't touch on their own lives. I have respect and admiration for people with that type of background who go through schools and get themselves an education. I'm lucky that I didn't have to fight for an education. As it is, I know enough to realize how little I know about many things.

I was fortunate enough to come from a literate and aware household. Dinnertime was devoted to talk, not formally about any one subject, but more time was spent on national and international events than on personal happenings. My parents were liberal, probably radical for their day. Our library had *Das Kapital*, in German as well as in English, and when I was grown and went about with a paperback Homer in my pocket, I realized I was probably unconsciously copying my father, only he read it in Greek. My mother was an early suffragette and a pacifist. If this all sounds serious, it wasn't. There were certain standards of decorum which we were expected to observe, but there was always a good deal of lighthearted teasing and a habit of bad puns which persists in the family.

When I was a youngster, my sister would go off to school, my father start for work, I'd have my breakfast, and my mother would still be sleeping or asking for her coffee to be brought to her while she looked over the paper and started her telephoning. I would be reading. I read the usual boys' books, and then read my sister's versions of Nancy Drew, or whatever little girls read in those days, including Louisa M. Alcott and the Little Colonel series. I went through the usual children's books in a hurry, outgrowing Tom Swift and the Rover Boys quite early and moving on to more adult books. There was a large library of classics and current literature in our living-room bookshelves, and our children's bedrooms had their own bookcases. At one period, I practically lived in *The Book of Knowledge,* just as at a later time, downstairs, I lost myself in the *Britannica.* My memories of *The Book of Knowledge* made a request from its editors a few years ago particularly interesting. They wanted me to supply them with some information on a subject about which I'd written a book.

At any rate, I do not remember being bored or unhappy when I was home alone when others of my age were off at school. I was brought up, too, with Robert Louis Stevenson's *Child's Garden of Verses,* and the world was "so full of a number of things . . ." When the weather was good, as mentioned, my mother took me on a long (in time) walk every morning. We would leave as soon as possible after ten and, if there was time, walk to the corner and back before lunch. Walking that slowly, I was forced to develop habits of observation that remain with me. I've been told I'm observant, which I always credited to good eyesight until I realized that some of it came from training. Having to occupy my mind with the happenings in the same locale day after day, I had to make them more interesting because the scenery passed so slowly. So I trained myself to notice small things, the differences that come about with the seasons, changes taking place or being planned in houses and grounds. Those early walks could have been a bore, but they never were to me. What they were to my mother, I hate to think, but she remembers them today with pleasure. She was involved with watching my progress or lack of it; I was busy trying to walk.

I think the main purpose of these walks was to give some muscular activity to my legs, although because of the way I moved, practically every muscle in my body got a workout. And they started in me something else not usually realized by people without mobility handicaps—the constant scrutiny of the terrain. Even my mother, who helped me develop it, has forgotten about it, and she, and others, will point out a roughness in the pavement or a potential hazard, without realizing that I have automatically seen it, noted it, and taken it into account. People with me rarely realize this because I do not seem to look down while walking.

This habit of noticing the ambience came in handy later when I became a small-boat sailor off the coast of Maine, and when I took up flying. It seems perfectly natural for me to be watching at all times to see what's coming up. It is also one of the reasons I'm a good driver (I think). In the city or on the road, I automatically look ahead for possible difficulties. When I was the editor of some automotive magazines, I discovered that most successful racing drivers have that trait built into (or beaten into) their systems. Generally speaking, when driving you shouldn't have to bang on the brakes or use your horn often; almost all driving emergencies can be foreseen.

I remember that when I was quite young I was terrified of dogs, large or small. I think that was a reasonable fear. I was very unsteady on my feet, and a neighbor's exuberantly affectionate pet might easily have knocked me down. It may have been that, or it may have been caused by a neighborhood dog rushing out and growling fiercely. This happens often—many dogs will growl or bark at a person walking with crutches. I suppose it is some kind of fear they have of a man with a stick. I'm accustomed to it, though it embarrasses my hosts if it happens at a home where I'm not a regular visitor and thus known to the dog. Usually, the commotion subsides once I sit down and put away my crutches, but some animals that may have had unhappy experiences, or guilt feelings, will growl or bark every time I move.

At any rate, when I was younger and less steady, dogs were a minor problem for me. So my sensible parents got me a puppy. It was a very small poodle of toy size when full-grown, which he wasn't the day he appeared. He must have weighed all of two pounds and was as terrified of me as I was of him. I shut us up in the back hall, where we had a stand-off, or in this case it might have been termed a sit-off. I didn't want to get too near him, he didn't want to get near me at all. The little back hall had one wall, doors leading to the front hall and to the kitchen, both doors now closed, and a stairway leading to the back hall on the second floor. I sat on the bottom step, and if the puppy got up the nerve or curiosity to approach me, I would scoot backward up a step or two, which he was too small to climb. We spent that afternoon getting acquainted that way, and in time I realized he was more afraid of me than I was of him. That was the end of my fear of dogs. No one said to me, "We're going to get you a dog so you will get over your fear." They just gave me a puppy as a present and let nature take its course.

That was so long ago his name was Tip, short for Tipperary, which it was a long way to in the British song of World War I. I don't know what happened to him or how long he lived with us, and my mother's diaries don't mention his passing. I do remember that he was eventually replaced by the dog with which I grew up, a gentle, old-fashioned collie that loved me the way a collie traditionally loves a child. I say old-fashioned because these dogs had been a working breed.

Later, they became fashionable in America and their appearance changed. They were bred for show purposes, with
longer and more pointed noses. I've always thought the
newer ones were more nervous, due to inbreeding, and that
their narrower heads contained less brains, which is probably
untrue.

Her home name was an unoriginal Queenie, and she was
a huge animal, brown, white, and black, an integral part of
my growing up. And a part of the household until I went
away to college. She missed me so much that she was given
away to friends who had a large farm complete with sheep,
so she could end her life taking care of them as she'd been
bred to do. Like any dog, she was often in a hurry, to chase
a cat or another dog off her territory, or check on the credentials of a visitor. But I cannot recall that she ever bumped into
me or even brushed against me when I was standing, even
when she was expressing her joy at my returning after an
absence of ten minutes or two months. She was always gentle
with me, but, with the sensitivity of a pet, seemed to know
when I'd just had an operation or something that would
make me particularly vulnerable, and at such times she
wouldn't get rough or too close even when I was sitting or
lying down.

She was a living part of my life for eight or ten years, an
important period in my development, just as my Irish Mail
was a mechanical part of my life for a few years. For the
benefit of those who have forgotten or never knew, an Irish
Mail was a four-wheeled vehicle that had a seat in between
the four wheels, propelled by a handle that the rider pushed
back and forth, and steered by the rider pushing his feet one
way or the other against a front axle that pivoted. Somehow,
my parents found a fancy Irish Mail I could use. Instead of
being a bar, the handle that provided the motive power was

a wheel, which also did the steering, so I could use it without needing any leg muscles. In addition, it had a gearshift of sorts: in the rear position you had power, provided by moving the driving wheel back and forth; in the center position, you were in neutral so you could coast; when you pushed the gearshift lever all the way forward, you had a friction brake.

This was important to me as a child, the way an automobile was later, because it gave me mobility, independent mobility. When the other kids were out playing on their bicycles or skates, I could be with them on my Irish Mail. It couldn't go everywhere they could, or as fast, but it provided me with a way of being a part of their activities.

From the time I was very young, we had a car and a chauffeur. My mother drove, but my father never did. Either my mother or the chauffeur drove me around. I never had a wheelchair for use at home, except for short periods when I was recovering from an operation. My father was a medium-sized man with wide shoulders and a strong back. And an even stronger character. I remember him carrying me on his back so I could participate in many things I might have missed or have been too tired to appreciate—art museums, ball parks, zoos, theaters, and the like. Fortunately for my development, both my parents had a wide range of interests.

I was in and out of schools and hospitals until I was thirteen and in the second year at a large public high school named Soldan. Every morning, the chauffeur drove me there in time for the nine o'clock classes and then returned to the house to drive my father all or part of the way downtown to work. Having a brilliant and studious older sister precede me at the school was a mild disadvantage. Teachers remembered her and expected me to be as good. This was made worse by an aged Latin teacher who had taught my mother and some uncles—by all accounts except hers, mediocre students at best. But because my sister was studious and hard-working, she remembered them as having been fine students, so she threw their mythical exemplary work at me and expected me to equal her memory of them. I didn't.

I was bright enough to do better than I did, but I was also lazy. I had read too much, and was a little bored, I think, with having to read things I had gone far beyond, and in some classes trying to catch up in fields where my preliminary training and drill were lacking. I had developed a bad habit that stayed with me in college: I depended too much on what I knew and on my ingenuity, and studied just hard enough to get by. I had a horrible confidence that I could pass any examination, and I did often enough to make me think I always could.

I don't remember too much about high school. I know I was driven to school a little early so I wouldn't have to enter in a crowd. I was allowed to leave my classes a couple of minutes early so I could get to the next class without being caught in a mob. For the same reason, I was picked up by the chauffeur a few minutes before the final bell. Without my parents' knowledge or approval, he would drive directly to the park and get out of the car so I could slide over to the driver's seat, and I would drive to within a few blocks of our house, when we would reverse the process. In this way, I learned to drive so that when I grew old enough to be allowed to do so, I would know how. Long before I started doing that, I knew I would have to figure out my own system for driving a car while using only one leg. I had worked it out in my mind, but I had to find out whether it would work in practice.

By the time I got to college, I knew there were some things I could do and some I couldn't. In order to be involved in some form of athletics, I went out for the rifle team. I made the freshman team and won my numerals, and the following year won a major letter in a minor sport, by a freak. I wasn't that good. I was, say, the sixth man on a five-man team, a general substitute. But we won the Eastern Intercollegiate team championship that year and, by custom, were thereby entitled to major letters. Only one of the required positions was "standing." I was not as steady as a rock in that position, and my "standing" scores varied from the barely acceptable to the just plain terrible, but my sitting, kneeling, and prone scores were good enough. After my sophomore year, I dropped out of the rifle team. I wasn't that interested in it as a sport and I thought I had made my point. I was entitled to wear a big white sweater with a large blue "C" on the chest, the kind of thing that goes home with you, ends up in a trunk, and eventually gets lost.

A few years later, when we were living in a small town in southern Illinois, bowling suddenly became popular again. I watched a few times, but by nature am not cut out to be a perpetual scorekeeper. So I asked the proprietor to put up a small handle on the lefthand wall of the lane on the extreme left, to enable me to have something to hold on to and steady myself while I bowled with my right hand. It worked well enough. I never became very good, but I wasn't a drawback to the team on which I played. I suppose that was the main reason for my athletic attempts, a matter of pride, of not wanting to be singled out or pitied.

As a kid, when you went to a new place, a new school or summer resort or whatever, you were a curiosity for a time. Kids are at one and the same time kindly and considerate and thoughtless and cruel. So are adults, often with less excuse. It was important to me to be able to participate. Football would never be my game, almost by definition, but I could participate in a way in backyard baseball and basketball.

Baseball I played mostly on my knees, sometimes as a pitcher, sometimes as a very tied-to-the-bag first baseman. I didn't have any range, but my arms were always long and strong, and I had good fast hands. As a batter, I was at best mediocre, and when I hit the ball, someone ran for me. In basketball, I played a sort of stationary forward, and in time developed a pretty fair set shot. These things sound minor, but they were important to me at the time, and looking back, I can see why.

For a couple of years in my earliest teens, I went to a summer camp in Maine, very advanced in that era, as it was not rigidly programmed with important, inflexible schedules. In this camp, the children chose their own programs, each one making up his own mind about what he wanted to do. It was a camp that didn't emphasize organized team sports, but stressed individuality and personal actions. Horseback riding was one of its features, something for which I was about as unfitted as I was for the high hurdles. But I was a good long-distance swimmer, and at my best in a canoe, where arms and torso strength are more important than legs. To gain some kind of water-sports award, a camper had to show his skill by, among other things, "walking" the gunwales of a canoe. As this was obviously beyond my capability, I did it by walking the gunwales on my hands. I was surprised then, and am now, that this was noticed as a feat. It seemed so obvious to me: I couldn't use my feet and legs to do this, so I used my arms and hands. I had a peculiar advantage as a swimmer: the bulk of my weight was above the waist, and I discovered early in life that with my large chest I couldn't sink. In fact, to swim underwater, I had to keep moving fast, aimed down at a sharp angle. I also learned to sail at camp, in sailing canoes. Later, when I had a series of small sailboats on the coast of Maine, I realized that learning to sail in a canoe gives you a pretty good grounding in the basic principles and fundamentals, a feeling of respect for what wind and water can do, and a certain amount of confidence in your ability to withstand them if you treat them with care. Just as the knowledge that you can't sink gives you a certain confidence when on, in, or under the water.

Swimming reminds me of a nasty trick I used to pull. I have always had a dislike for what I call "old ladies" of either sex, usually sentimental elderly females. Strange ones used to stop me on the street and infuriate and humiliate me, though they weren't smart enough to realize that, by saying, "What a shame you're not a girl with all that lovely curly hair." When you're a little boy, it's terrible to be told you should have been a girl, and it was worse to know that these old ladies were trying to say something they thought would be nice because they felt sorry for you. When you're young enough, anyone over thirty-five is old enough to be an old lady.

When I was growing up in St. Louis, we used to go away for the summer to various summer resorts, to the mountains, the northern woods, or the seashore. No matter where they were, there was a certain pattern to these resorts, and also to the people who went to them. The typical summer places centered on a big house, stone or wooden, surrounded by cottages for guests with large families. On seashore, lake, or mountain, they all had a spacious front porch, usually wooden, where the old ladies sat and rocked and talked and kept their eyes on other guests. At this period, my dislike of old ladies was fully formed, and once a year, or more often if the audience changed, I would get my revenge.

I would go out to the swimming float, which was always within view of the front porch, put my crutches down on the diving board, and seemingly fall off, landing in the water with a splash. I had to do this soon after we arrived, before the old ladies realized I was quite capable of taking care of myself once I was in the water. I would stay underwater for a time and come up on the far side of the float, so people on the porch couldn't see that I was breathing air instead of inhaling water. Usually, someone would become alarmed enough to send down a spotter to make sure I hadn't drowned, by which time I would be plainly visible and just an innocent swimmer. I'm not proud of that trick—it wasn't at all nice of me. On the other hand, I'm not as ashamed of it as I should be.

I used to play another game that seemed to arouse the old ladies, but that was only a by-product. I had a good friend on the block, a boy named Lee, very tall, very blond, and very quiet, a gentle soul if there ever was one. We used to go places together, and as we walked I would try to trip him by sticking a crutch between his legs and he would try to kick a crutch out from under me. It was a game that was more of a threat than anything else—I don't think I ever tripped him or he ever made me fall. But, once every so often, some "old lady" would see us and recognize one or both of us and telephone Lee's mother or mine. These had to be strangers because anyone who knew Lee would know he had no malice or meanness in him. Usually, the callers complained about his treatment of me, but sometimes they objected to both of us behaving in this ungentlemanly fashion. My mother, who knew about our little game, would politely thank them and tell them to mind their own business; Lee's mother, whom I liked and who, I think, liked me, would say she would speak to us about it.

Looking back on my childhood, I realize that a part of my good fortune was in having been incapacitated very early, so I had a chance to get accustomed to my limitations. The fact that I had a generally equable temperament was also just plain good fortune, though some of it may have been the result of training. Because many things were discouraging or painful or impossible, I realized when I was quite young that I couldn't dwell on them without making myself unhappy.

Children are generally conformists among other children. Each one wants to do what the others are doing, even if it's whitewashing Tom Sawyer's fence. There were times when a little group of kids would start to plan something that I couldn't do. Rather than make it obvious, I would make an excuse to get away from the group, if necessary inventing something that I had to do right away. I thought at the time that I was doing this to spare their feelings, so they wouldn't feel guilty about excluding me. Now I wonder whether it wasn't a form of self-protection—whether I didn't get away from the group so I wouldn't be left out, thus making it obvious to everyone, and particularly to me, that I was different.

Physical activities are more important when you're young than they are afterward. I learned quite early that there were a number of things I couldn't do, and I suppose I had to learn certain forms of self-discipline so I wouldn't spend too much time being unhappy. Some of the things I had to learn as a child are still a part of my character. I'm normally a friendly and gregarious soul, but I had to spend so much of my youth alone or without young company that to this day I not only don't mind being alone, I rather like it.

I become impatient with people who get bored easily. There are so many things I want to know, to learn about, and to do, that I have little sympathy with people who always have to be entertained. I am not a "group" person and tend to stay away from large parties or other large gatherings. I live and work in New York and have family in St. Louis and often drive the thousand miles between the two cities. I would rather drive it alone than with a companion, except for a few individuals. Despite what might be thought of as a stand-offish attitude, I would say I've always been popular. I had never thought about my own popularity until I began to work on this book. When I stopped to think about it, however, I realized it was something about which I'd never been concerned. In my conceit, I always took it for granted that I would be liked and accepted wherever I went, despite what might be considered an ineradicable difference. And because I don't mind being alone, I always figure I'd be able to get along anywhere.

I'm not aggressive, socially or otherwise, but I've always been independent, not changing my views in order to be in accord with others. This is, I think, a little more difficult for a handicapped person, because it is adding a social or philosophical difference to an already existing physical one, and just about everyone wants to be popular and the easy way to achieve that is to agree. But while conforming can and does make things easier, you have to be sure you don't conform at the expense of what you consider your principles and ideals.

One of the troubles with having a physical handicap is that, being different from most people, you are always noticed, whether or not you want to be. So, as a rule, anything you can do that lets you fit in without being set apart is grist for your mill. One mild exception to this, when I was young, was that I started wearing long pants earlier than the usual age. This made me look different, but it also hid the fact that I was wearing braces and that my legs were so thin. I still remember going to school in a state of mild trepidation, wearing my first pair of long pants. At my first class, I sat next to a big redheaded boy, a star athlete of the future. As I sat down, he clapped me on the back and said, "Welcome to the big leagues." It was nothing but a small, friendly gesture, but it made me feel good all day.

Although you may not be expected to do many physical things, for obvious reasons, many people expect a person with a physical handicap to be smart, and to be more ethical than others. This got me into trouble once, in college, when I'd cut a class to take my girl friend (later my first wife) to Annapolis for a crew race. It was a beautiful weekend, but when I returned to school, I was greeted by friends who told me I'd gotten into trouble while away. I had cut my one Saturday class, in chemistry, and the professor, seeing a very small class, unexpectedly took attendance by handing out three-by-five cards, asking the students to write their names on them and answer a small, simple question. It was the first really nice warm weekend of the spring, and there were a large number of absentees. Also a large number of cards. The size of the stack of cards evidently was disproportionate to the size of the class, or rather to the number of people there that day. The professor gathered the cards and read each name aloud, looking for the owner. Many of the names must have belonged to ghosts, as there were no bodies.

According to reports, he was shocked when he came to my name and there was no answer. The others in the same situation he just put into a different pile, but he reportedly came back to mine and made some remark. At any rate, I was called in, lectured, and then asked who had filled out the card for me. I said I didn't know and was threatened with being expelled after being reported to the Dean, etc. It hung over my head for a week or more. Fortunately, my best friend's father was head of a linked department. He knew and out-ranked my angry professor, and he went to bat for me, and the whole thing quieted down. My friend's father, I later discovered, was somewhat shocked that my professor had become so vindictive about a small matter—not that I had cut a class, but that I wouldn't say who had filled out a card for me. Although I wouldn't say I knew who had done it, he might have figured his son knew, but he didn't ask either of us. The thing is, out of maybe twenty absentees whose cards showed up, I was singled out for harsh punishment for no reason that I could imagine except that I walked on crutches, and while I was being lectured, the professor said, "I expected better from you."

There are a lot of things you can't do with a motor disability; almost anything that requires much moving around can be a vocational handicap, even though your disability wouldn't interfere with the performance of your work. Early in World War II, I realized my conscience wouldn't let me stay home and write fiction. As I had studied engineering in college, I applied for work at several war plants, and got turned down every time. Finally, I went to one of the major plants where I knew one of the owners, who called a department head with a recommendation, and I still wasn't hired. Later, I found out why. It was feared that in the big, busy, cluttered plant and its type of precision work, my handicap would raise the insurance rate.

Actually, it was a matter of timing. The big war industries thought they would be able to keep their key help. When someone sent me to see someone I knew at the newly formed Office of War Information, I was welcomed with open arms, and as soon as I could be cleared, I went to work as a junior news writer in the New York office of the Overseas Branch. Within a year or so, many of the firms that hadn't been interested in me discovered that they wouldn't be able to keep many of their key employees and I was flooded with offers, as I was obviously a legitimate 4-F and would never be called up. Despite this, when there was Congressional fear that government work had become a haven for draft dodgers, I was called in for another physical examination.

Because I had no idea of working for the government permanently, I did all the things an ambitious civil servant wouldn't do. I volunteered for responsibilities no one else wanted, I stuck my neck out, fought with my superiors, and committed the unpardonable sin of making decisions on my own. When I did this, by pure dumb luck, the decision proved to be the correct one. As a result, I moved ahead faster than anyone I knew in the organization, and ended up very high on the ladder. While I sent hundreds, possibly thousands, of people overseas, I was never able to go myself. Because of my physical condition, it was felt that I could become too much of a responsibility. I gave my month's notice the day the war ended, and, to my surprise, six months later was back in government, working for the Department of State.

One of the troubles with a physical handicap like mine is that you are not only identifiable but apt to be remembered. I have a very good memory for certain things and a terrible one for names and faces. As a result, I am constantly greeted by people I realize I should know, and I try to get a clue to their identities by thinking back to how I knew them. My work for the government, where I had been the supervisor of perhaps ten thousand people, was no help to me that way; it complicated my problem. I always blamed my poor memory for names on the fact that I was so easy to remember because I was identifiable. But one day, many years after leaving college, I was stopped on the street by a familiar-looking man who was a former classmate and friend. We made a date for lunch later and renewed our friendship, which continues to this day. But at lunch, as we got ready to leave and I reached for my crutches, he pointed to them and said, "You didn't use those in college, did you?" I had to start right then finding a new excuse for my inability to recognize people. I haven't found one. I can't even blame my age, as I've always had this problem, which I can only call a form of stupidity.

CHAPTER THREE

Be Proud of Yourself

Telling someone to be proud of himself sounds like the oddest of admonitions. Pride of the wrong kind has caused a good deal of trouble in the world. But pride in one's self is important for everyone, and particularly so for the handicapped. Words and terms change; like styles of dress, they go in and out of fashion. Today, psychiatrists, psychologists, and amateur advice-givers talk about ego strength. Young people talk about finding out who they are, and of identity crises. This is nothing new—the young have always had that problem. It just seems new, and it is probably more difficult today, as the world moves faster now, changes are more rapid, and there are many more people. So there are more people to learn about, more people who will have to discover and label their own identities and to find what their places in the world are or will be. The problems aren't new, only the terms describing them are.

A person with a handicap may have more of an identity crisis than one without. He also may have an advantage, an unusual one: he is accustomed to having to fight for things, and he knows what he is fighting against. I have come to the conclusion, along with a few experts in the field of working with the handicapped, that the main effect of a handicap on an individual's personality is to amplify or emphasize characteristics that would have shown up anyway. The timid become shyer, the bold become more aggressive. As I've said, I don't think that suffering ennobles. It can make people bitter, but it seems more likely to give the bitter sufferer a rationale for being bitter; it may seem to make the Job-like character more patient, but probably it gives him a theater in which to show his patience; it works the same way with the reverse situation, allowing the short-tempered to show their impatience.

Being proud of yourself is important, because people are often treated as they think they should be treated. The handicapped person has to be conscious of himself as an individual, a personality, a worthwhile human being. This isn't always easy, as some of the handicapped think of themselves as useless because there are certain things they cannot do. That doesn't make a person worthless except in his own eyes, which is where the chief danger lies. The world often takes a man at his own valuation, if he is downgrading himself. The converse is not always true. If a man considers himself superior and isn't, the world will take a certain amount of pleasure in beating the conceit out of him. For the handicapped, it should be a matter of sensible analysis. In analyzing his good and bad points, he can find reasons to be proud of himself for his strong points and build them up, and at the same time try to alleviate what he considers his weaknesses.

I am no person to speak of this. To the best of my knowledge, I have never made any deliberate effort to improve myself. I've gone into things that have had that effect, but any such result was accidental. I was evidently born with a large bump of curiosity, so that I like to find out about things, almost everything. Often I've been able to, which has resulted in a possibly unwarranted sense of self-confidence. Someone once said to me, "You licked a physical handicap, so you think you can do anything."

That's a mistaken judgment in several ways. In the first place, you don't lick a physical handicap, you learn to beat it down, to make it bearable, to cope with it so that you run it and it doesn't run you. I don't think I can do anything, only that I can do a number of things unthinking people wouldn't expect me to be able to do. And I think that if I want to do something reasonable badly enough, I will find a way to do it. The whole trick to this is to stop and analyze the problem, to figure out why you can't do it with your particular disability—and then to figure out a way it can be done. Most of the things I've really wanted to do, I've been able to do. Not always well, not always at once.

Every time you are able to do this, it adds to your confidence, which makes it easier next time. And, every time, it adds to your belief in yourself, something everyone must have in order to lead a moderately happy life. Sometimes the obstacle is a familiar one, bearing a relationship to one that has been surmounted in the past; sometimes it seems to be completely different, but the fact that you've overcome previous problems seems to make this one simpler. Mainly, success of this type comes from experience in overcoming obstacles, and this is something the physically handicapped know a good deal about.

I have considered that having a physical handicap has been an advantage in certain ways. Not that I would recommend it, but it forces you to think in certain ways. I have been the editor of a number of magazines, of a newspaper feature syndicate, and I've run a large news room. These are fields in which it hasn't been necessary to run or move about very spryly. Because I was unable to run, my experience has taught me to shy away from being impulsive about doing anything important. As a result, my working judgment has been considered good. Naturally, I've made mistakes, too. Sometimes by being too cautious, missing an opportunity while pulling back to consider things from all angles. Sometimes because I was too confident that I could do something that turned out to be impossible, at least for me or my organization. **1799183**

Being cautious or taking chances in business or in a profession goes along with doing the same thing physically. In each case, I suppose it becomes a matter of weighing the risks or comparing the possible gains. In a physical way, I know I have become more cautious as I've grown older. I have an old friend, an elderly man I have known for many years, whom I never visited because his apartment was up two very bad flights. It was just understood that he'd come to my place or we'd meet downstairs. But, a few years ago, he got very sick and couldn't negotiate the stairs himself, so I went to see him. It had become important for me to go up those stairs, so I sat down and pushed myself up backward, a step at a time, a method of climbing stairs I'd learned as a child when I didn't get around as well as I do now. The point I'm trying to make is I wouldn't have done something so undignified if he had been able to go up the stairs with me—it would have been embarrassing to him and to me. But paying this call was more important to me than possible surprise or pity from onlookers.

A fine line has to be drawn between being brave and adventurous, doing the things you want to do for yourself, and being foolhardy—and doing things so that no one will notice or realize that you are unable to do them easily. Just as there is a fine line between being proud of yourself and being conceited, or between being sure of yourself and being pompous. Almost everyone wants to be accepted and liked. For a person with a physical handicap, this can become an obsession.

There are a number of phrases used about the handicapped, generally recognized character traits that are attributed to them, or to some. Terms such as the "cheerful cripple," the "obliging cripple," or the "bitter cripple." They are all true of certain types, we've all seen them and met them, just as there are cheerful or bitter people of all types. Even the use of the word "cripple" is a thing—very few handicapped people use it in general conversation, as it has a pejorative ring. In baseball, a batter "hits the cripple," which is a 3–2 or 3–1 pitch that the pitcher has to make good or put the batter on base. The handicapped or crippled are more apt to use it about and among themselves than the general public is in their presence.

In a less sensitive day, when gradations of wording were not given the attention they get today, the word was used much more. There was a fine hospital in New York, The Hospital for the Ruptured and Crippled. In time it became The Hospital for the Crippled and Disabled, and now is just as fine a hospital under the name The Hospital for Special Surgery. Various institutions with the word "cripple" in their names have changed them. The use of euphemisms doesn't change the situation, but it makes it sound better to some and less offensive to others. Just as the poor or ignorant have become the underprivileged or neglected, the word "cripple" today is very rarely used to describe a person's physical condition. I cannot speak for the real feelings of others, I can only say that for me it is just another word. Despite its current lack of popularity, it has a certain validity when used as a noun with a preceding descriptive word. The "cheerful cripple" mentioned above is usually a person who does not have much real pride in himself or belief in his own worth and hides that fact under a false air of good humor. It is almost always pleasant to meet a genuinely cheerful person, but the "cheerful cripple" is a type it is no fun to be with for long. One soon discovers that his rather frenetic good humor is put on to disguise his fear of not being accepted or liked, or to hide his bitterness.

I know a rather severely disabled man who falls into this category. I was told by friends, "Oh, you'll like him, always in good humor." And, at first meeting, I did like him. Then I spent several hours with him and discovered that under his jovial, outgoing manner there was a strong streak of bitterness, that he wore a façade of good humor to hide his resentment of a world that had treated him unfairly. Not all "cheerful cripples" put on a mask to hide bitterness, but enough of them do to make the bitter cheery ones a recognizable type. A psychiatrist I had known socially for many years told me she had finally given up on trying to locate my hidden anger at the world. As I didn't know she had been searching for it, I was surprised. She had decided that I couldn't possibly be as accepting of what had happened to me as I seemed, so I must be hiding a deep resentment. I was not a patient of hers, but a friend and neighbor whose behavior or demeanor obviously didn't fit into the pattern she had selected for me.

Any attempt to classify people on the basis of outward characteristics necessarily runs the risk of error. The "bitter cripple" is more apt to be showing his true self, whereas the "obliging cripple" is usually, like the cheerful one, hiding his true feelings because he wants to be liked and accepted at all costs. These are people with physical problems who do not have enough pride in their worth to "stand up and be counted," to use an unfortunate phrase. I had been aware of many of these types because I have spent more time in hospitals and orthopedists' and physical therapists' offices than most people, and hearing them described as types caused me briefly to wonder whether I fell into one of these categories. I decided I might be considered one of the "obliging" type, because I am soft-spoken and not easily roused to anger. I might also be one of the "cheerful cripples" except that those who know me realize that my general air of good cheer is genuine. I don't mean by this that I never get "down," but most of the time I feel cheerful. This may be, like having an equable temperament, something for which I was trained or trained myself, in which case the discipline went on for so long that the cheerfulness became second or first nature. But I think I was just born to be what was described in song, by another man with that disposition, as "a cockeyed optimist."

This, of course, can be a matter of semantics. An optimist will call himself one, whereas a pessimist will not use the word "pessimist" for himself—he will think of himself and describe himself as a realist. I think that most handicapped people become realists—they have to—but only a few become pessimists. There are times in anyone's life when he has a sensible right to be pessimistic, times when things go wrong, and we know from experience that these times seem to crowd together—enough things will go wrong in half a day to take care of the bad luck for a week or a month. That is the way things go, in streaks or spells. At such times, I think the handicapped, who have had experience with real adversity, are less apt to get into a blue funk than most people. This matter of having pride in yourself goes along with a certain amount of optimism rather than a pessimistic outlook. Pessimism says something like: Things are terrible and they're going to stay that way or get worse. A person who has overcome problems and troubles is apt to think: Things are terrible, but I can overcome the worst of them—I have to.

Almost everyone with a halfway decent mind can find something about which he can be proud, some ability or abilities that can be developed. One of the troubles with people whose physical handicaps came upon them when they were young is that during youth the important things are usually physical, and the handicapped person discovers that the things on which his peers set a high value are apt to be things he cannot do at all or cannot do well. This makes it hard for him to feel proud of himself. What he can do to develop proficiency in something on which his age group sets a high value depends on the nature of his handicap. It also depends in a way on his ingenuity in persuading his group that certain activities in which he cannot excel are unimportant, whereas some things he does well are fascinating. If this sounds competitive, it is. We all live in a competitive world to some extent; children, with less experience than older people, are more apt to place high values on competitive skills.

In my case, it was fairly simple, a matter of mobility. Despite my powerful arms, I was never going to be good at climbing trees—legs are necessary for that. But there was nothing to prevent me from being good at marbles or mumblety-peg, games that are generally played with the participants on the ground. In a day before wash-and-wear and drip-dry, I must have been hell on clothes. I still am. Normal activities today have my crutches wearing out shirts and jackets under the arms. I like flannels and soft woolens, but I don't buy them because I wear them out too fast. When I was a kid, my activities on the ground wore out my trousers at the seat and at the knees.

Because it was important to me, I learned to be pretty

good at some activities in which lack of mobility wasn't important, and I soon realized that a child with a handicap had to be better than average at an activity in order to be accepted without question, to be chosen for any team without condescension. When I later took up golf, I knew I would never be a long-ball hitter, but there was nothing to prevent me from being excellent at approach shots and putting. These things could be developed with a good deal of practice, so I worked out a style of play to fit my capabilities: my "long" game was a series of shots designed to keep me out of trouble, to keep me on the fairway until I was close enough to the green so I could make up a stroke or two by skillful approaches and putts. My game broke down completely when my putting was off and my approaches weren't going close to the cup. Everyone's golf game breaks down when that happens, but other golfers' scores wouldn't balloon the way mine did, because they always had a chance to recover with an exceptionally good drive or long iron shot.

The person with a physical handicap has to contend with the fact that he must be above average in a physical skill to be considered adequate, and to realize that he will be expected to be above average in other ways. In a peculiarly reverse fashion, people who don't think much about these things, who really wouldn't want you on their side if the game involved physical activity even if it were something you could perform well, tend to think of you as bright or smart. You may not be any good at the type of "war game" boys play, because such games usually are based on speed and strength, but it will be assumed that you will be very good on the plans board, devising strategy.

This, of course, depends on the physical impairment. People who don't know any better think that certain types of illness that leave handicaps must automatically affect the sufferer's mental ability. I couldn't walk well, but that was obvious. If I'd been afflicted in a different way, so that my movements were jerky or uncoordinated, or my speech was slurred or indistinct, I might have had the mind of an Einstein and they would have considered me mentally handicapped. In their reverse way, because I had a walking difficulty, they wouldn't hesitate to ask me for advice about taxes or spelling or the state of the world.

I suppose that, in a way, I responded to this, sometimes negatively. I felt I had to know how to do anything that didn't take mobility. At a fairly early age, I learned how to play bridge, poker, chess, and other games. Not necessarily well, but well enough to get along in most circumstances. I remember that, when I was quite young, a chess-playing child prodigy from Europe came to St. Louis, where he gave some exhibitions, playing a dozen or more adults simultaneously. Someone who was involved with his trip thought I would be a good companion for him in his spare time, so we spent many daytime hours together for a few days. I wasn't thrilled. His English was slight and his interest was chess, so we'd meet and have little to talk about. He would want to play pool, a game at which I could beat him easily. So he'd suggest some chess, where he would wipe me out in a few moves or minutes.

I was not yet in my teens, but I knew that he had to find some way to get back his ego. The fact that I couldn't run or walk but could still beat him at a physical game like pool was most difficult for him to accept. Today he is a grand master, and if we should play chess, he'd beat me worse than when we were kids. And probably beat me at the pool table as well.

I never felt it was my social duty to be good at many of these games and pastimes, but I believed it was an asset to be able to play almost all games, to know their basics, just as

I have always felt it a plus to be able to talk to people in many fields with more than an amateur's knowledge of their profession or interest. Part of that was luck, part was due to my oversized bump of curiosity, which may or may not have been helped along by the hours I had to spend alone and reading. I know I discovered that the more you know about more things, the more you realize the extent of your ignorance and the number of things there are to look into and learn.

Practically everyone has some characteristics or traits with which he is dissatisfied. No intelligent person should be totally pleased with the way he acts or looks or the amount or depth of his knowledge or his social graces. If he is satisfied with himself, he is either stupid or smug, or both. A person with a physical handicap has additional factors with which he must contend. This makes it more difficult for him to build up enough pride in himself to be a whole, rounded individual.

According to Robert Louis Stevenson's outmoded lines, as the world is so full of a number of things, we should all be as happy as kings. There are many more things in the world than when he wrote that, and many fewer kings, and as communications improve and we are able to know more about conditions, few people would admit to being more than temporarily content. That is not because things are that much worse than they always were, it's that we learn very quickly today about people in the next city or county without enough food or shelter, and about people in countries thousands of miles away being killed or mistreated in some way.

The handicapped have more reason than others to be happy or unhappy, depending on their attitudes and circumstances. I put those two words in what I consider the proper order because the well-being of the handicapped depends so much more on how they look upon themselves and their problems than upon their affliction—as in the much-quoted lines about the two men who looked out between the bars, one seeing the mud, the other the stars.

One of the reasons some of the physically handicapped have trouble being proud of themselves is that they experience more frustrations than most people, and have to live with them. Recurrent frustrations, or a long series of them, can lead to violence, discouragement, or apathy, or all three, not necessarily in that order. Most people with a motorskeletal handicap become accustomed to it and do not expect the frustrations caused by it to be magically overcome or removed. Trying to be honest and objective, I cannot say that being unable to walk properly, or run, or climb, has been a frustrating experience, it was just a condition that came upon me. Certain things were and would always be impossible for me, and that was that. But one specific frustration could drive me up the wall, could make me edgy, irritable, and tense. A frustration caused by an impossibility is one thing, but when you can *almost* do something, that is a real and difficult frustration.

Many years ago, in the medical attempt to make my almost useless right leg a useful member of my body, I had an operation or two that were a series of muscle transplants. Weak or useless muscles were replaced by stronger muscles that were not so necessary in their original locations. This was not a comfortable process, but the pain was not the most bothersome part of it. The main trouble came from nerve actions and the brain and connections to it.

The question was how to get the brain accustomed to the new locations and functions of these old muscles, and how to get them to respond to commands that are normally not directed by a conscious portion of the mind. It is a maddening experience to issue a command for a muscle to perform in a certain manner and then to have the command ignored. How do you get it to work? This is not something that anyone else can do for you, you have to work it out yourself. It is discouraging and almost impossible to believe when your conscious mind says to raise your leg and nothing happens. You can sit in a chair day after day and tell your leg to straighten out, to kick, and watch it hang there with no more response than you'd get from ordering the earth to stop revolving.

That is difficult and discouraging but not as frustrating as the feeling that comes when you get a transplanted muscle to obey a command . . . once. It does it once and won't do it again. You try to figure out how you got it to work that one time, you try to play back every step of your thought processes. How did it happen? Why won't it do it again? Your brain tells you that it is a nerve connection, that a new pathway has to be created, and a word like "synapse" comes to mind. You know what it is you're trying to do, you know the effect you want to get. But just exactly what do you have to do in order to get the muscle to respond?

Sometimes, after the first proper response, you don't get another one for days or weeks. You know that you can get the muscle to work if you can only issue the proper order in the right way, because you did it once. And then, one day, you do it again, and after a few more days or weeks you are able to do it almost at will. In due time, the new channel for your nerve path from brain to muscle becomes established, and eventually it becomes routine and the switch takes place from conscious to automatic. But before that, the period when you know the response is possible but it won't answer to your command is about as frustrating as any experience a person can have. It is much more of a problem than merely being unable to do something you would like to do. It is a most annoying experience, because overcoming that frustration is not a feat from which you gain any satisfaction. I have felt a sense of accomplishment when doing something that I felt was helping to get me over an obstacle that was preventing me from leading a normal life. But this was just getting a muscle to do what it was supposed to do, made difficult by the fact that it had been transplanted. Normally, getting our bodies to perform certain functions or activities is not a problem. In most circumstances, we breathe, see, talk, hear, and go through the motions necessary to live and get through the day without giving them a thought.

This points up one of the differences the handicapped learn to live with—the fact that certain things that seem to be routine for the "normal" person can be done by the handicapped only if he concentrates on them. Each type of handicap has its own problems that way, and not only each type but each handicapped person. No outsider can know what is or will be easy, difficult, or impossible for a handicapped person, because, though the handicap may be obvious and can be fitted into a general category, each individual's reaction to it will be different.

Occasionally, we learn a new skill—how to type or speak a new language. As we gradually master the process, we feel a certain pride of accomplishment; even if we're not doing it well, we think we'll do better as we go along. We can be proud of ourselves, in a small way, for that.

But that is a different kind of thing, and is not what I meant when I said that it was necessary for a handicapped person to be proud of himself. Not because he feels he can do some or many things better than another person—that is a different and dangerous kind of pride. You have to be proud of yourself as an individual, because you are unique. Not because you have been favored by nature so that you can do things better or faster than others—that is usually false pride. The number of "fastest guns in the West" who found out fatally that they weren't helped raise those stupid, sad statistics. But no one else is exactly you. Maybe you don't always like what you are or the way others may see you, but you're still you and no one else. No other person has a combination of genes and molecules and atoms arranged just the way yours are. This should be a source of pride for you. If it isn't, you have to work to make it so, or you'll be one of those unhappy people who make everyone around them unhappy because they are unhappy, who are disliked because they don't like themselves.

CHAPTER FOUR

Compensate— Don't Overcompensate

A person with a handicap has to make up for it somehow. For his own sake or because he thinks he has to in order to change the way others regard him.

Most people act as they do because they are conscious of the way their actions may look to the rest of the world. No one lives in a vacuum, we all react to the reactions of others. Too many people with handicaps downgrade themselves. The admonition to be proud of yourself is a counter to putting too low a valuation on your worth. It is probably worse to pay too much attention to the way others may regard you than to pay too little. As is true of almost any behavior, moderation is the best policy.

We're all familiar with the Little Napoleon type—the short person, male or female, who is so conscious of his lack of height that he tries to make up for it by pushing other people around. With some people, the worry about their size is physical; with others, the fear is of a lack of mental stature and they try to make up for it by arrogance, cockiness, or brashness. The touchy, inflated ego of the physically or mentally undersized is a good example of the type of overcompensation often indulged in by the handicapped.

I have seen it in many, and have often wondered whether I don't fall victim to it, too. Because I have physical weaknesses that are apparent, I think I may try to give the impression that I am stronger, tougher, or braver than I am. One way I often do this is by a refusal to admit weariness. As a result, I have developed stamina, partly by refusing to give in to exhaustion. I know this is often stupid—you can get a lot done that way, but you can also reach a point where neither your body nor your mind is performing properly, and you should learn to call a halt before that point is reached.

In the same way, it is common for a physically handicapped person to try to do something that his handicap makes difficult or impossible for him. That, often a matter of overcompensation, has to be balanced with the idea that if the handicapped didn't try to do some of the things that seemed to be impossible for them, they would never stretch or reach their capability horizons.

Twice, I have come upon people who walked slowly and with great difficulty being used as messengers. It struck me as a stupid and inefficient use of their bodies, so, butting into things that were none of my business, I inquired. One messenger was the physically and mentally handicapped younger brother of a large family, and it was the only way they could use him, they said. They also told me that he felt better being able to contribute something to the family business. The other case was what I can call mistaken philanthropy by a notably unphilanthropic firm. He had applied for a job and that was the only one they could find for him; rather than turn him down, they had put him into an unsuitable post. He was in it for ten years before the firm went out of business.

In neither case had the handicapped person tried to get into the unsuitable type of work. But the handicapped often do, according to some personnel managers, who say it often puts them into an awkward position. And I've discovered that what might look like an unsuitable job for a person may not be. I asked one personnel man about a man with a bad limp working in the shipping department. "He can do the work," the personnel chief said. "It bothers me to watch him, but it doesn't bother him to do it. I've offered to move him and he rejects the idea. He explained that he doesn't read too well or too fast, and it makes him nervous if he has to. The work on this job is primarily physical, the amount of reading he has to do is minimal. He became upset when I asked him twice about moving him. He wants to stay where he is, and the important thing is for him to have a job in which he is comfortable."

I had started by wondering whether the husky-looking man with a limp hauling those heavy crates around was over-compensating. He was obviously proud of the fact that, despite appearances, he was doing the type of work he was doing. He might have considered it giving in to a weakness to have worked to learn to read better so he could take what would seem to be a more suitable job. Whether or not it seemed to be overcompensation, he was working and he was happy at it. As I had discovered before, outsiders, whether they're well informed or ignorant, well intentioned or just meddlesome, can never tell about any individual handicapped person.

Anyone with a physical handicap has learned how to manage and has had to learn to keep his body pretty much under control. Which brings up the matter of alcohol and drugs, two major methods in our society by which people with handicaps, usually emotional ones, try to compensate.

I have heard many stories of alcoholism among the handicapped. Like the story of Mark Twain's death, they are exaggerated. That doesn't mean alcoholism doesn't exist; it does. There are enough handicapped people who add alcoholism to their other handicaps to give a certain factual basis to the stories about the high percentage of drunken handicapped. From everything I could find out about the subject, that isn't a true picture.

Whether you view alcoholism as a physical illness, a mental illness, a problem of heredity, or a lack of willpower, it exists and it causes a tremendous amount of trouble. I'm not going into possible causes or cures—I'll leave that to the experts who have been differing on various phases of it for years. All I'm concerned with at the moment is alcoholism and the physically handicapped.

To start with, I'm not talking about someone who takes a drink occasionally or regularly, or who goes off on a binge once every so often. I'm perfectly willing to use the old Alcoholics Anonymous definition of an alcoholic: a person who can't take *one* drink. In other words, someone to whom an excess consumption of alcohol is a problem, whose drinking interferes with the regular conduct of his life, professionally or socially.

Drug addicts and alcoholics have at least one thing in common: to hear them, it is never their fault. Their families, their friends, their government, society didn't treat them right and forced them to become addicted as an anodyne. Many alcoholics say they don't like the taste of the liquids they force down their throats; some main-lining addicts say they are afraid of the needle. In their reasoning, this shows that they were forced into it.

Let's take up alcoholism first. Despite the horrifying stories I've run into, my own investigation has convinced me that alcoholism is not a major problem to the handicapped.

The handicapped have a built-in excuse for becoming alcoholics. They are often in pain physically; they are often in pain psychologically because of some of the things that make them different from the unhandicapped; they are often frustrated because their physical condition doesn't allow them to do all the things they want to do, the things that others do. Alcohol looks like a way out. Who could blame them if they drank too much? Who would cast the first stone?

Nevertheless, the percentage of alcoholics and heavy drinkers is lower among the handicapped than among the rest of the population. I've heard one reason given repeatedly by nondrinking handicapped people and by ex-alcoholic handicapped. I can understand it because I feel the same way. Much of my working life has been spent with hard-drinking people. Most of my friends and associates have been connected with communications: newspapermen, advertising people, entertainers. I have done a good deal of heavy drinking and have never been drunk because I have a built-in stop. A doctor once said to me, "You have to keep yourself in shape. For you, getting around at all is an athletic feat."

Some former alcoholics among the handicapped have said the same thing: "I stopped because I couldn't handle it, and I have enough trouble getting around when I'm sober." Others have said that if they drink too much and can't handle themselves, it makes them dependent on other people. These are things the nonhandicapped rarely think about, but I know it is one of the reasons I don't get drunk. I've spent too much time and energy fighting to be socially independent to do something that puts me into the hands of others. As a result, there comes a point, no matter how uninhibited the festivities, when I put the brakes on my intake. I have no hard-and-fast rules, no set amount of drinks at which I stop —I just slow down after a certain point. One of my excuses to myself is that I am usually driving. It is one of the reasons that I prefer doing the driving to being driven—I know I'm not going to get drunk. This whole matter of not drinking to excess is not something I ever decided, it just worked out that way. I knew I couldn't afford to get drunk—I'm wobbly enough when sober. As a result, drinking has never been a problem to me. I've never depended on liquor except as a mild social icebreaker; it has never occurred to me to take a drink by myself.

That "never" I have to modify, like Gilbert's Captain of the *Pinafore,* to "hardly ever." The number of times are so few that I can remember the incidents. Once was during World War II when I held a somewhat responsible and sensitive position with the government. I was in charge of a department and at the time was working on the overnight shift, which meant that I got to my desk some time before midnight. A few minutes before I was to leave the house, I received a phone call that my kid brother, a pilot, had been killed. On the way to work, I decided I wasn't going to mention this to my co-workers, and I stopped at a bar and had a couple of quick drinks.

The only other time I can remember going into a bar by myself and getting a drink was also connected with a death. I received a phone call that my father-in-law had been found dead in his apartment. His daughter, my wife, was in Mexico and his son was in Canada. I had to go to the morgue to identify for the police a body that had been dead for a few days and was no longer in good shape. That night, after finally reaching my wife and telling her, and talking to my brother-in-law, I went to a lively café and had a meal and a few drinks.

It was a perfectly respectable place, but not the kind of bar or restaurant I would have gone into in normal circumstances. I was using liquor then as a mind-deadener. I was upset by the circumstances of the death of a man I had liked. And upset for his daughter and son, and I wanted to rid myself of the picture of that decomposing face. But generally I stay away from drink except for purely social purposes. Liquor has been called the glass crutch. It doesn't seem to mix well with wooden or aluminum ones.

In addition to my built-in controls, addiction to alcohol or drugs has never been a problem for me. I didn't feel I had any need for them; my life was full enough—I had too many things to do. But it is easy to see how the stories of the handicapped being large users of alcohol or narcotics could crop up. Both are pain-killers and dream-makers, a way to escape reality, and the handicapped may find the reality of their afflictions hard or impossible to bear. It is easy to see how they could turn to either to get them through a bad period and then let it become a habit. But it doesn't happen very often.

There aren't many statistics on the subject. A British study was made during World War II of the use of drugs by hospital inmates. It was found, to no one's surprise, that those in the hospital with permanent disabilities used no more drugs than the others, but those whose disabilities were incurred during or because of air raids showed a marked increase in the use of opiates (up 100 percent) during or immediately after air raids. A few days after the most recent raid, however, their demand dropped to normal. An American Veterans Administration doctor said the use of drugs or addiction was not considered one of the major problems among veterans until the Vietnam war, when the percentages went up all over the country, among the able-bodied as well as the disabled, who seemed no more addicted than the hale.

In fact, he said, it might be lower among the disabled, for the same reason that I heard given often about alcoholics among the disabled: most people with mobility problems had no desire to make their moving around any more difficult. While the use of alcohol or drugs by the handicapped would be a form of compensation, the overuse would be a definite form of overcompensation.

I have seen the fear of addiction to either become a factor with the handicapped. I know a man with a bad limp from one cause who will not take a drink because his hands are not steady for another reason. I had noticed that he wouldn't drink when we were eating in a restaurant. He had explained privately that he was afraid of making a spectacle of himself. Once, at his house, he offered me a drink and I noticed he didn't take one, though he poured me one. I asked him if he never drank, and he said very rarely. I asked him whether he found it made his shaky hands worse, and he said it didn't seem to, so I dropped the subject. I had no desire to talk anyone into drinking.

I have heard tales of people who became addicted after having been introduced to drugs while in hospitals, but I have not been able to verify these stories. These are people who have been given opiates as pain-killers and later, according to the stories, were hooked. It is possible that this happens. I have never seen it. But I have seen instances where fear of possible drug addiction has caused what seemed to be unnecessary problems for patients.

One of these took place in Boston when I was still young enough to be in the Children's Hospital. My doctor was operating on two patients, of whom I was one. The operations

were about the same, as much as any two corrective operations can be the same. The other patient was about my age,
had a similar medical history, and seemed to be a bright kid,
cheerful and healthy except that he had been crippled by the
aftereffects of polio. I was operated on a day before he was.

I started before he did and was ahead of him all the way.
Not by just one day. After the first few days of recovery, one
day's difference will be absorbed. But my recovery was so
much speedier than his that I began to wonder. I finally asked
a floor nurse whether we hadn't had about the same surgery,
because it seemed to me that I was much more comfortable
than my friend, and making better progress. She said it
seemed that way, but when I wanted to know why, I received what I considered evasive answers.

The question remained with me for some time, until I was
able to ask the doctor about it. I had not imagined it, my
recovery was much speedier, my discomfort had been less.
I had been receiving pain-killing drugs, in gradually decreas-
ing amounts from the time of the operation; the other boy
had not, because his parents objected. They were afraid that
he would become accustomed to the comfort of drugs and
wouldn't be able to do without them later. "Because they
were afraid," I said, "he went through a lot of pain that I
avoided. And because of that, my recovery was much faster."

The doctor nodded and we got into a discussion of the
connection between pain and the rate of recovery. He made
me formulate a theory that after an operation the body
needed all the strength it could muster to get itself in shape,
and fighting pain used energy that might better have been
spent building up the body.

Some years later, I had a related experience with a roommate in a semiprivate room in a New York hospital. In this
case, the roommate, a year or two older than I, was having

a hard time, taking no opiates after his operation because he was afraid of becoming addicted. We were both adults, so I could discuss it with him. The avoidance of the pain-killers was his idea. His mother, a widow, came around often, distressed because he was obviously in pain. She pleaded with him to take the medications prescribed for him, but he refused to take any opiates. When I asked him why, he told me he wasn't going to get any drug habit. I said that I thought that was ridiculous, and he accused me of being an addict and wanting to get him addicted, too, and acting as a stooge for his mother.

I'm not saying his reaction was a normal one, but I had no way of talking him out of it. He suffered—unnecessarily, I think—and I was glad to leave him when I was able to go home. I thought the two people mentioned, afraid to take drugs because of a fear of becoming addicted to them, were behaving in an irrational manner, but I am what might be termed a non-pill-popper. The only thing I take regularly is saccharin. I like coffee and tea, and I like it sweet, and I don't want to add the weight I might gain with sugar.

I'm no sylph, being short and stocky, with wide shoulders, long arms, and a thick chest, which upper torso development probably came from moving myself around by my arms for many years. It was feared that I might get fat after I had polio, as I had a normally healthy child's appetite but couldn't get the amount of exercise that most growing children do. So I grew up eating very few fats or starches. As I grew older, this became a habit. I don't have the usual desire for forbidden fruits, don't even like most of them. My mother is no cook, but even if she were, Mom's apple pie, or any pie, is not my idea of heaven. To me, a good meal consists of lean meat or fish, broiled, not fried, and lots of green vegetables and salad. My consumption of potatoes, pastry, or bread, except in an occasional sandwich, is minimal. What surprises me is not that I don't eat these things but that I don't want them.

A couple of years ago, when I had an emergency cholecys-tectomy, I was a mild disappointment to my doctors. Most of the things I was supposed to cut out or cut down on for a time after my gall bladder had been removed were things I didn't consume anyway. I don't drink much, I stopped smoking a few years ago, and I stay away from fats or fatty foods. Some of the handicapped are grossly overweight, partly from the difficulty of exercising, often from the difficulty of exercising willpower about eating. Many people, frustrated by things they cannot do or have, compensate by over-eating; it is more noticeable among the handicapped because they do not have the same opportunities to work off the excess calories.

I'm not at all sure that some of my activities—not at the dining table—are not forms of compensation for physical handicaps. My interest and work in sports, for instance. If I couldn't do them, it gave me an excuse to watch them and become an expert in some of them. This may be true of many of my interests—my curiosity about almost everything may be a form of compensation because there are many things I can't do. I think my interest in aviation is, and was, legitimate and quite normal. But learning how to fly may have been nothing but an attempt to overcompensate for not being able to walk properly, and being too earthbound. Maybe being able to look down on forests was my way of making up for the trees I was unable to climb as a child. I'm not sorry that I did it, because it added to my total knowledge and experience, and I enjoyed it.

I think I overcompensate in other ways. I mentioned that I will rarely admit to being tired. I consciously try to minimize pain. Some people have thought I was brave because of that, but I know better—I know I'm a coward and am afraid of pain. And I have enough imagination to be able to see it coming. On the other hand, trying not to show it, not to give in to it, has sometimes caused me unnecessary trouble. I remember being quite uncomfortable after one operation. I had expected to be—when you go in for a complicated operation, you know it will hurt. But there seemed to me to be a good deal of surface pain connected with one area during my early recuperative period. After a time, when they changed bandages or removed a drain or something, they discovered that I was quite raw near the wound. Someone had used the wrong material and I was chided for not having called it to their attention. My explanation that I had expected it to hurt and didn't want to complain wasn't really understood.

Without acting like a martyr, a handicapped person can compensate by not whining or being a complainer. Logically, a person with a physical handicap can be a burden to others. There are things he cannot do, there are times when he won't be able to pull his own weight, so to speak, so he shouldn't add to the burden his presence may cause for others by complaining about his lot in life. He can compensate, in effect, by being considerate. In a group, he can volunteer for something he can do that no one else wants to do; he can avoid advocating any form of group activity in which he might need the assistance of others due to his singular condition.

When I started thinking about doing this book, I had a few questions to ask my mother, as she was the only person who might know the answers. One of the main questions in my mind was whether it had been a conscious effort on the part of my parents to raise me to lead as normal a life as possible rather than turn me into a "brilliant cripple," which might have been possible when I was young. Not that I was so smart, but people often thought I was, being deceived by the fact that I wasn't exactly inarticulate and had done a tremendous amount of reading very early in life.

Her answer was that she couldn't recall that at any time it was a deliberate choice, something she and my father had talked over and decided. But they had realized when I was quite young that they weren't going to have to worry about my mind. Parents have a tendency to think their children are smarter than they really are—or dumber. So, without discussing it or making a project of it, they bent their efforts toward enabling me to lead as normal a life as possible. To a certain extent, I cooperated. I think I shied away from the "brilliant cripple" concept quite deliberately. One of my classmates at some school walked very badly and was a limping portrait of the "greasy grind." He was considered a genius, and was usually alone and looking unhappy. Every time I saw him that way, I said to myself: There but for the grace of God go I. Of course, he might have been the same if he had walked perfectly normally. I know that I did no more work than necessary to get by. My grades were mediocre—fortunately for me, it was the era of the "gentleman's C"—but I knew a lot of my fellow students, and was involved in all kinds of activities, not all of them involved with my formal education.

Even the university was fooled about my intellectual capability, and I was allowed to take twenty-two points a semester, when sixteen was normal and gave you enough points to be graduated on schedule. As a result, I was enabled to take many courses that had nothing at all to do with my supposed goal. I was studying engineering, with the idea of becoming an aeronautical engineer. But with all the points I was allowed, I was able to take many courses in literature that otherwise I would have missed, plus others in history and psychology. Sometimes I took them because of the subject, sometimes because of the person who taught them. In one of these, I studied under the late Mark Van Doren and was very much impressed by his combination of intelligence and sensitivity, as was everyone. I had no way of knowing then that he and his wife, Dorothy, would later become so important to me and my first wife. But I wonder, now, whether taking courses in medieval history or Russian drama or economic geography was a part of my curiosity or a form of compensation.

I was never a big wheel in campus politics, nor did I try to be, but I was a definite part of the little group that more or less ran the class, possibly the only one of the group who was neither an athlete nor a fraternity member. I was surprised recently, when forced by this book to think about the past, to realize that most of the leaders in the class today, as alumni, were also leaders when they were undergraduates. What I ask myself is: Was I involved in all these things—politics (local and national, not campus), sports, the arts, friendships and activities off-campus—as a compensation for not being able to run or walk? Or was it a conscious or subconscious desire to round myself out?

Which brings up that whole subject. The happiest handicapped people I know are those with the greatest number of interests. Come to think of it, the word "handicapped" can be omitted. But as the book is about the handicapped, perhaps it had better remain. I know a few able-bodied people who have only one overriding interest but seem quite happy. They happen to be outstanding in their fields, and the single-minded happy ones I can think of, as I said, are few. Most leaders in specific fields who seem content or happy in their outside lives also seem to have an unusually large range of interests.

According to current social historians, the greatest problem most people face after they get by the basic one of survival is loneliness, a lack of communication. This is something that becomes more noticeable and more important with advancing age. The similarity of the problems of the physically handicapped and the elderly becomes more apparent with age, until the two blend into one, in many cases, and being old becomes a handicap. This matter of loneliness and lack of communication with others is one of the simplest and least desirable things for the handicapped to achieve. They are less apt to be doing things in a crowd, they are apt to meet fewer people, they are therefore apt to know or be friendly with fewer people.

One of the things in my favor is that I have never been lonely, or perhaps was too stupid to realize it. I'm a moderately sociable and gregarious person. I find people fascinating (except in large groups) and so many different things interesting. But because I had to spend much time by myself when I was young, I grew accustomed to falling back on my own resources, and that is why I get impatient with people who complain about being bored when alone.

What I'm saying is simple and basic: the more you do, the more you want to do. And the more things you do, the more interests you have, the more people you're apt to know. Popularity, mere numbers of acquaintances, is not a worthwhile goal. But the more interests you have, the more different things you will be able to discuss in an interesting and knowledgeable manner, the more people will be interested in you.

For a realistic belief in your own worth, you have to have some confirmation. The fact that other people find you interesting is an indication of your individuality and the strength of your personality. Psychologists use terms like "ego" or "ego strength" for something everyone needs to be a successful, functioning human being. But the handicapped person needs it more than others; his handicap is a long-lasting or continuous assault on his ego, on his dignity as a person. To repel this attack, he needs an extra portion of ego strength. I use this term rather than plain "ego" as we have a tendency to confuse ego with egotism. What is needed is not conceit, which is putting too high a value on yourself, but a realistic appraisal of your own worth.

Practically everyone, whether or not he will admit it, wants to be popular. The well-adjusted person will acknowledge this if he is forced to think about it; otherwise it doesn't enter his consciousness very often. It is not difficult to be popular without having to be a sycophant to every outsider's key likes and biases. All that is necessary is to have a genuine interest in other people and in subjects that are not necessarily connected with your own life. A key word in that sentence is "genuine" because a pretended interest eventually shows its falseness. Being involved in enough different topics makes more people interesting to you and, reciprocally, you to them.

It is very easy for anyone who is in any way different from the general run of people, and particularly for the handicapped who are externally and noticeably different, to retire into a self-absorbed internal life. This is another point of similarity with the aged, who often do the same thing. It is dangerous to do this. Not for the world, just for the individual who does it. Much of the time a person with a physical handicap spends at a doctor's office or a clinic is devoted to answering questions about his physical or mental state. If nothing else, this attention paid to his condition forces him to think about himself. And it is easy to confuse the medical attention paid to his condition with a personal one. He can easily fall into a frame of mind in which he thinks everyone is interested in his physical condition.

This is true of almost everyone who gets sick, and is understandable and can be a mildly amusing foible ("Would you like to hear about my operation?") when a sudden, unexpected, or spectacular ailment comes up. It is not the same when the condition is chronic. Then it becomes a bore. Which is, or should be, the last thing anyone with a handicap wants to be. The way to avoid this is to compensate—by being interested in other things, other people.

CHAPTER FIVE

Pity

Pity, like sympathy and akin to it, is a recognizable and legitimate human emotion. Any person who can look at another's suffering and not be moved by it in some way is not a complete human being. This, of course, is one reason why, in a war, the enemy has to be seen as a different kind of being. We can't purposely destroy and inflict pain on others like ourselves. Our enemies have to be Chinks, or Commies, or Gooks. They're different, and the difference has to be accentuated. Being different, they can't have the same feelings and emotions we have, so we're not really hurting them so much. Historically, after a war, we mask our guilts by providing necessities, amenities we've been careful to take away while we were fighting, things like food and shelter and medical supplies.

The handicapped in our society are also different. They

will receive a certain amount of sympathy for their afflictions, which is normal. They will also receive a certain amount of pity that in time most will come to hate or relish, depending on the individual. Pity can work more than one way, for both the giver and the recipient. The pity that comes from the idea of a fellow human less fortunate than the viewer and goes on to a desire to help improve his lot in some way is one thing. The pity that comes from the fear of being like the one pitied is something else. Pity from an outsider can be constructive or destructive; helpful or damaging.

Probably the worst thing that can happen to a handicapped person is for him to feel sorry for himself. This can be the most damaging result of an accident or illness or birth defect, because it is almost sure to stop any serious attempt at rehabilitation. Self-pity, while understandable in many cases, is the most totally negative and self-destructive emotion in which a handicapped person can indulge himself.

As is true of so many things, that is true of the able-bodied as well as of the handicapped. However, I see it from the point of view of a handicapped person who is trying to improve himself, to battle against the physical conditions that can hold him back. While self-pity can be as great a drawback for the nonhandicapped, it is not as obvious, and while it can also keep him from improving himself or reaching a life of fulfillment, that is a totally different story.

We've all known people who feel sorry for themselves, with or without reason. Some poor souls are always in that state, and are truly to be pitied because, no matter what happens, they will remain wretchedly unhappy. Most self-pitiers feel sorry for themselves only at intervals, when their psyches are at a low state for some reason or other. These people will proclaim, and many of them honestly believe, that no one has ever had it so bad, has ever been so put upon, has ever had so many bad breaks, has ever had to put up with so many wicked people who had it in for them for no reason. Their cry is the same, their plaint just like that of the self-pitying handicapped: Why did this happen to me of all people? Why was I singled out, why was I so chosen, what did I ever do to deserve this?

It is easy to see how anyone who has been deprived of the use of any of his faculties can feel sorry for himself. A little boy or girl, or a grown man or woman, seeing others do things he can't do and would like to do or even be able to do, can easily wonder: Why me? If a person is born with a handicap or acquires it early, he is apt to become accustomed to it and learn how to cope with it. A person whose capabilities have been drastically changed by an illness or accident is more likely to have a hard time finding an answer to that "Why me?" question. A question that becomes the ultimate in self-pity, a question that is a call for attention, that is saying, in effect: Look what happened to me! Isn't it terrible? If you had any decency at all, you would feel almost as sorry for me as I do for myself!

I've known handicapped people who feel that way, some of them bitterly and openly, some hiding it. I've talked to many of them, trying to talk them out of it, generally with no success.

Probably the most interesting thing about people is the fact that no two are alike. But, in many respects, the self-pitiers are much alike, whether male or female. You have the feeling that if you've talked to one, you've spoken to them all. They are envious of those who have escaped their problems and difficulties. They don't take any of it in if you point out to them the difficulties and problems that other people have. They don't want to think that anyone could be worse off.

That would destroy the rationale for their self-pity, that they have been specifically selected by a malignant fate to be the goat for many of the world's ills or misdeeds. I have a theory, never tested, never proven, that people have inherent limits to their capacity for feeling—for enjoyment or suffering or worry. Most of them worry or suffer or enjoy to the limit of that capacity, regardless of the worth of the cause of that feeling. These seem to be patterns that rarely change, though I once saw a rather dramatic change.

I had been in a hospital, and while convalescing spent part of an afternoon, at an official's invitation, in Children's Surgical, and had come away, as I usually did, filled with admiration for the courage and cheer of the kids. I spent part of that evening with a middle-aged man who was recovering from a conventional, not too serious operation. He spent a good deal of time telling me of his problems and troubles. They didn't seem that serious to me and I probably wasn't as sympathetic as he wanted me to be. I'd known this man for some time and he always felt that he was abused, unappreciated, and generally unlucky, that everyone else had it better than he did.

Some time after that, his condition in life changed drastically and inside of a few months he was no longer among the privileged. For the first time in his life, he was thrown into intimate contact with people whose worries and problems were basic—whether they would have enough food for themselves and their children, and a roof over their heads. This man did a complete turnabout. Instead of seeing everything from the standpoint of how it affected him, how it was directed by an unjust Nemesis to make life difficult for him, he saw that other people had problems that made his look insignificant. To his credit, his attitude about himself changed. In time, his economic situation changed for the better, and I'm sorry to say that he reverted to his former self-pitying state.

Anyone, handicapped or not, who feels sorry for himself—

with or without reason—is in a terrible state. But a handicapped person burdened with self-pity is in a worse condition, because it means that he is without the one prop that
keeps most of us going: hope.

A handicapped person who has fallen prey to self-pity for
more than the briefest periods and has given in to the luxury
of despair will stay that way as long as his main feeling is
being sorry for himself, because that attitude will keep him
from making the effort necessary to improve himself and his
condition.

I was horrified and discouraged once to meet a man I'd
known earlier who had become a victim of self-pity. I had
met him when we were both children going to Dr. Robert
Lovett in Boston. Let's say his name was Bill Grey, which it
wasn't. He lived in a nice suburb of New York on Long Island,
and after we met at the doctor's we became friendly and so
did our families. As we grew older, we saw each other less,
but I was invited to his home for an occasional weekend
when I was in college. Then we lost contact with each other
for many years. I finished college and moved back to the
Midwest, and when I came back to live in New York, I didn't
think about him. A number of years had passed, I was married and had a couple of children, and he was a small portion
of a distant past.

After a lapse of many years, I received a phone call from
him and we made a date for lunch a few days later. It turned
into a traumatic experience, certainly for me, probably for
him. The last time I had seen him, he had been a busy, vital
young man. He had had polio, as I had. Now, that is, or was,
a nasty disease whose aftereffects vary with each case, but it
is not a wasting, progressive disease. It does its damage and
leaves you, to recover or not; it does not get worse, year after
year, as some diseases do. Once it has done its damage, it

leaves you alone, wrecked, unaffected, mildly affected, or reclaimable.

At one time in our joint careers, Bill had been in better shape than I. His family was wealthy and had spared no expense. I remember that he had a car equipped with various hand controls. I didn't. I also remember that his family's house, a three-story home rather like the one in which I had grown up, had a small elevator built in, to take him from the ground floor to the second, or on up to his den on the third floor. I thought of both of these things because they had been topics of discussion at my home, talks in which I took part. I didn't see any reasons for them, for me. I had worked out a way to drive, using the standard controls of the day on a regular car, and it had worked out all right.

As for the stairs in my house, they were something to which I had become accustomed. I went up and down quite often. I didn't go up and down them without a thought if I'd forgotten something minor, but they were a part of living and my life. By agreement, I rarely used the big front staircase, which was wide, curving, and decorative. I used the back stairs, which were narrower and had a ninety-degree turn at a landing. I either scooted up and down on my rear end, or hung on to the railing on one side and pressed against the wall on the other. The mahogany railing on the front stairs was a beautiful thing to slide down, but too wide to be easily graspable to help me climb, and my often dirty hands would have left a mark on the light papered wall. My hands did the same on the backstairs wall, but it was plastered and painted brown and could be washed, and no one saw it except the household help. About my hands, I might add that I don't have a Lady Macbeth complex, but anyone who uses his hands as much as I do for getting around finds he has to wash them constantly to keep from leaving spots.

The last time I had visited Bill at his house, he had been involved in various projects connected with his school and community. He seemed to have many friends and to be a leader in his little group. I had rather liked and admired him, particularly his drive and seeming zest for life.

I drove to the restaurant we had chosen, reserved a table, as he didn't seem to be there, and sat at the bar and had a drink, watching the late-coming lunchers. Finally my lunch date arrived, being pushed in a wheelchair by an attendant. Trying to hide my shock, I got up to greet him and guide him to the table. The bright, vital young man I had known had been replaced by a washed-out, gray old man. I don't mean his hair was gray, *he* was gray, with the drab lack of color one finds in a long-term convict.

I will never be on any list of the best-dressed men because I'm not interested in fashion. I dress to suit myself, wanting only to have enough clean clothes to wear. But I was shocked at Bill's appearance. At a time before it was fashionable for men to wear long hair, his hair was long and messy, and looked as though it hadn't been washed for a long time. His clothes were old and dirty, not with the look of poverty but messy with a look of neglect and lack of any care or consideration. Seated next to Bill, I looked like a fashion plate.

I don't remember whether or not he had a drink, but he was evidently a fussy eater, as he gave the waiter full details about the dishes he ordered, which surprised me a little. I have a theory, possibly because I am easy-going, that the physically handicapped who have adjusted to their condition aren't overly picky. My theory is based on the idea that their experience with pain and illness teaches them the difference between what is important and vital and what is not worth bothering about. So I was surprised to see Bill fussing over his food even before he had received any. It also didn't fit in with my memory of him. At his house, we had lunched hastily on a couple of hamburgers, over his mother's objections, because we had too many things to do and talk about to spend time going to the dining room for a regular lunch.

We started talking, rather stiffly and with difficulty. Our lives, which had seemingly been somewhat similar when we'd met before, had become completely different. We were like two trains that had run on parallel tracks for a time and then had come to a switch point and gone on in different directions. We tried without success to find subjects on which we could talk easily. He asked a few questions and I asked a few and we both discovered that, despite a somewhat common past, we had less to share than almost any two strangers who might meet at random.

I found out fairly quickly that he had never married, that he lived alone except for a man who waited on him, and was obviously something of a recluse. He seemed to have no close ties and was noncommittal when I asked about his brothers. He mentioned that his father was dead. I noticed that he did not say his parents, only that his father had died a few years earlier, so I asked about his mother and he said she was dead, too. I also noticed that, though he'd been given the opportunity, he didn't ask about my parents, whom he had known. By this time, I had come to the conclusion that he was now a self-centered and rather ingrown man.

I had stopped volunteering information because of the obvious disparity in our ways of living. He asked whether I lived alone, which I do now but didn't at that time, and I explained that I had been married twice and had helped bring up four daughters. Instead of living alone, I was often surrounded by a spouse and a bunch of kids and their friends, dates, romances, etc., which I liked. Not the kind of thing you tell an obviously soured man who lives alone.

And then he asked me a question that hit me like a bullet. Trying to make conversation, I had asked him whether he had seen Dr. Ober lately, the onetime assistant to Dr. Lovett who had taken over his practice when Lovett died. Bill said not in many years. Had I? I said I went to Boston to see him on occasion, and he'd come to New York and operated on me a few years earlier. Bill gave me an odd look, and said, "Oh. You're still trying?"

It was less of a question than a statement, and it's difficult to describe the effect of that negative remark. I had been feeling sorry for him and his life, and wondering how we had taken such different paths. His statement made me see one of the reasons, or perhaps *the* reason. To me, trying is automatic. Not trying is a form of evil, or, if I believed in sin, sinful. To me, not trying is total nihilism. If you don't try, who is going to try for you?

I answered a brief yes. He asked how the operation had worked out and I said only fair, it had not been a complete success. He nodded as though to say what else could you expect? It had been a long, complicated, painful job, so long and complicated that it had been done in two installments, two weeks apart. I had been on the operating table for a good many hours, too long for one session since it wasn't an emergency. Besides, as I teased Dr. Ober, he wasn't as young as he had been once, either, and it might have worn him out, taken him almost as long to recuperate as it took me. But Bill Grey's comment brought that operation back to me and stuck with me. I was glad to leave him after lunch. I didn't hear from him or see him afterward.

I was puzzled by what had happened to him, and wasted a certain amount of time and energy looking up a few people who had known him, trying to find out why he had changed and unable to come to any conclusion. He had been thrown

by the death of his father, but that is something that happens
to almost everyone, and he was a grown man by that time.
If Bill had become that dependent on his father, then neither
of his parents could have done a very good job on him, or
with him. I kept trying to discover what had caused his
change, and discovered that he had died a few years after our
luncheon. I had the feeling that was what he had been waiting for.

His was not a usual case. In my experience, people rarely
change that way; their characters or characteristics are set at
an early age, and a fighter rarely becomes a quitter or vice
versa, unless outside factors bring latent characteristics to the
fore. I have seen that happen, but not with anyone who'd
battled a handicap since early childhood, only with those
who had been hit with adversity later in life and found it
more than they could handle.

But Bill had been fighting his problems for years, bravely
and cheerfully and, it had seemed, successfully. The last time
I saw him, it was obvious that his troubles had won. He had
given up. His question about me still trying was just an expression of this. It finally beat him completely, and he died.
I couldn't find out the cause of death—no one seemed to
remember. It wasn't anything spectacular, he had just died.
My feeling was that he no longer wanted to live badly
enough to put up a battle for it.

This isn't scientific, but I've found it true in too many cases.
A person's will to live cannot keep him alive in all circumstances, but, other things being equal, the most important
factor in keeping the seriously ill alive is their own strong
desire to live. Very few people can do what members of a
certain African tribe are supposed to be able to do: decide to
die and do it. But many people do it in a negative sense, by
giving up the battle for living. What had caused the once-

vital Bill Grey to give up, I'll never know. But something had happened to him in the years between our two last meetings; he had changed so dramatically that he felt sorry for himself.

This had become obvious during our luncheon conversation. He made mildly humorous, bitter remarks about his state. By this time, he was middle-aged, the world was against him, fate had turned him into a cripple, no one loved him. During a brief social lunch, I couldn't tell him that his disability had happened years ago, that when he was an adolescent, at a time when people take things hard, he had been leading an active life, he had liked himself well enough to project an attractive image. Now he was right in a way: no one liked him; he despised himself.

A reaction such as his is more apt to happen in a person who has been hit by physical misfortune after having become accustomed to leading a normal life. A person who has been a battler all his life, but not against a physical handicap of his own, may quit when he has to fight against an unexpected infirmity of his own. We expect a person we know is a battler to be a fighter in all fields, but that isn't necessarily so. A man I knew, liked, and admired, a man who had been brave physically and morally, fighting stubbornly against various forms of injustice for many years, amazed me by giving up completely when he was hit by a crippling injury. Within a year, he had died. A nonfatal injury had killed him because he couldn't summon the strength to fight against it, and without that strength he didn't care enough about living to stay alive. He would have fought with me if I'd told him he was committing suicide, but that, in effect, is what he did. The survival instinct is powerful, but it needs motivation.

I knew a case that worked out more happily. A woman who had borne up bravely under one cruel blow, who had rolled with the punch and made her adjustment, almost went un-

der when she was hit by another, years later. Of course, there
is always the so-called breaking point, the straw that breaks
the camel's back. But some people, like Job, seem to bear up
indefinitely, while others, surprisingly, buckle.

This woman, Susan, had had a hysterectomy when she was
still quite young. I met her because my first wife, Adeline,
had known her and went to see her. Adeline had had the
same operation when she was twenty-two, and knew it was
quite a blow for any woman at any time, and a particular one
for a young, newly married girl. We had decided then that
we would adopt children eventually, which we did. My wife
had discovered that the world was full of old wives' tales
about the effect her hysterectomy would have on her, on her
sex life, on her attractiveness, on her figure, on her personality. So, when she heard that a friend of her youth had had
such an operation, she went to see her, saying she would have
liked such a visit after her operation. The two women did not
live in the same area, but we made it a point to visit Susan
and her husband whenever we could. In due time, Susan
recovered from her depression and started making plans.
She was quite interested when we adopted two little girls, a
couple of years apart, and a few years later she did the same
thing, going us one better by adopting three.

Except for an exchange of Christmas cards with an occasional picture of the growing family, I quite lost touch with
her after Adeline died. Then I received a rather incoherent
letter from her, asking whether I could come to see her as she
couldn't travel to see me. I telephoned as soon as was practicable, and went to see her. She was living in a pleasant sub-
urban house, and greeted me from a couch on which she was
lying. Less than a year ago, she had lost a foot and the use of
one leg in an automobile accident.

Susan's comeback after her hysterectomy, with its upsetting psychological aftereffects, had shown she was a battler. But this seemingly lighter blow, the loss of a foot, appeared to be too much for her. She was perfectly content to be miserable, to play up her misery, lying in her bed or on a chaise and complaining. Her self-pity almost finished her. A "Why did this have to happen to me?" cry was understandable for a time, but it became a constant plaint. Hadn't she had enough to put up with? Why had she been so singled out?

There is no point trying to cheer up someone in a mood of that type. To point out that she had a loving, considerate, and understanding husband, was fortunate in being able to live as she did, had three lovely children and a host of devoted friends and relatives, would not have had any effect. She wanted something from me, something I wasn't able to give her: some words of wisdom or advice that would make her feel better, as though the end of the world hadn't come.

After a couple of visits, after I realized that I couldn't think of anything that would work, I told her the truth as I saw it: that she was pampering herself and enjoying it, that others didn't feel as sorry for her as she did for herself. The only surcease I could offer was that this was something she had to live through, for herself and the people around her who loved her, and that time would eventually come to her rescue, she would get over this and adjust to it.

I said it, but I wasn't sure. She was too wrapped in her own misery to have any thought for anything or anyone else. I spoke to her husband again and he told me something he hadn't mentioned before. She was complaining about the pain in her missing foot and had come to the conclusion that pain-killing drugs were ineffective, and had started putting away more and more brandy.

"Phantom pain," incidentally, is a common ailment. A missing member can, and often does, hurt just as though it were present, only more so. It can hurt, get too hot or too cold, get restless, and, worst of all, itch. This is a most difficult thing to deal with. It does not happen to everyone, and, as far as I know, there has been no definitive study to find out why it happens to some and not to others, why for some people it is so severe, for others minor, or even why those who suffer from it have it badly at some times and in a small way at others.

Phantom pain would seem to be semipsychic in origin, which doesn't make it hurt any less. A sharp pain in a part no longer connected to you sounds silly, but it isn't. Pain takes place in the brain, a response to a stimulus from nerves disturbed by something unusual. When there is an amputation, for instance, the nerves are disconnected along with the rest of the missing part. But at the other end the nerves are still connected to the brain, and any stimulus sent by them is felt as though it came from where the nerves had originally been located, not from the new place of origin. The poor, dumb brain is fooled, and telling yourself that your foot can't hurt because it isn't there any more is no more effective than telling yourself you're not seasick, the ocean isn't that rough.

Susan's phantom pain and her treatment for it and her total self-pity bothered me because I had admired her and was disappointed in her and didn't know what I could do for her. And then she was cured in an unexpected and spectacular way. One of her children got a "bug" of some kind and was rushed to the hospital with a very high and mysterious temperature. Susan was so upset that she forgot about herself. When the child recovered and came home, Susan was busy taking care of him and too grateful to feel sorry for herself, and after that she could hardly go back to her self-pitying pattern. Not only would no one believe the world was as hard on her as she had said, she couldn't even believe it herself. A child's serious illness had become a form of shock therapy.

But she had to have retained some of the elements of the fine woman we had liked before, or she wouldn't have reacted so violently to her child's illness. She would have given lip-service, but wouldn't have been so vitally concerned that it overrode all her other concerns, as indeed it should have.

Nothing I have come across has given me reason to change my feeling that self-pity is the most destructive emotion that anyone, handicapped or otherwise, can entertain.

CHAPTER SIX

Pain

Pain is a part of life—it enters into the consciousness of everyone. Unfortunately, the handicapped too often suffer, and have suffered, more than their share of pain. I'm speaking now of physical pain. The cause of their handicaps, an accident or a disease, was often painful and usually followed by more painful treatments. There is also the psychological pain of being different, of not being able to do all the things you want to do. That's a different kind of pain, sometimes harder to bear but not the same as a physical hurt.

One of man's benisons is that he is unable to recall pain accurately for any length of time. Talk to a woman who has recently had a painful childbirth (it does happen) and she will tell you, "Never again." A few years later she has usually buried the experience. A poet, Robinson Jeffers, said, "Pain is a thing that is glad to be forgotten." We don't know how well or how sharply animals remember pain, but physical punishment is one of the standard means used to train them, so they must be able to associate it with certain acts or forms of behavior. Physical pain, like most pleasures, takes place in the brain, not where we say it hurts. It is, in its way, a mental thing, as is love or beauty. There is, however, nothing good about pain. It can be useful or necessary, to show doctors the place or extent of trouble, but except for that, it is not easy for normal people to find a good word to say for it.

As is true of every other experience, pain is bound to leave its mark, to make an impression. Some handicapped people have faces that seem lined with pain, others do not. The ones whose faces don't show it are not necessarily those who have suffered less, they have just reacted differently. Pain is, like humor, very subjective. It is difficult to measure because the measurement cannot be objective. It cannot be measured with a light meter or a decibel counter, because it is a sensation—it has to be felt or it doesn't exist.

I have found that one of the best ways to live with pain is to know what's happening and why. Some people don't want to know. Some people get relief by yelling or making faces, others don't. I find that a pain you know is more bearable, possibly because you realize it will end sooner or later. Usually, I've been lucky in having doctors who understood my feelings about this and explained what they were doing.

I've been able to watch a certain amount of medical work being done on me. Some medical men object, saying that many people will imagine a worse pain if they can see what is happening. I remember being annoyed because I was crossed up once by a doctor. I had smashed my elbow in a fall, and my shattered bones were held together for a time by a metal pin. Eventually, after my arm was whole again, the pin began to cause trouble and had to be removed. This was a minor operation, performed under a local anesthetic, and my doctor had agreed that I could watch it being done. At the crucial moment, the doctor swung around so that all I could see was his back bent over to open my elbow. I protested, and he said, "Just a moment . . ." There was nothing I could do but stare at his white-coated back. In a moment or two, he stepped aside. All I could see then was a nurse putting a small bandage over a slight incision and a few stitches.

This has very little to do with pain, except that it was part of my theory that the more you know about what hurts and why, the less it hurts you. That is a theory that works . . . for me. I know it does not work for some others. I've seen them get sick at the idea. I've seen them flinch at the thought of pain, even of a pain they were currently suffering.

One of the difficulties of talking about pain is that it comes in so many different forms. The pain of a burn is different from that of a bruise, which is different from that of a cut, which is not like that of a headache, which doesn't resemble the feeling of a toothache. And there are different kinds of pain connected with every toothache or headache. A cut from a knife isn't the same as a paper cut. Etc. As pains differ, so do reactions to them. Some people reportedly have low or high thresholds of pain. Whether these differences are physiological or psychological is not easy to determine. Humans, however, have devoted a good deal of time and thought and ingenuity to finding new and better ways to inflict pain on others, usually for their own good, of course: to teach a lesson or to save souls, or to show the futility of resisting the pain-givers.

For many years, Western man seemed to feel that the inflicting of pain on others was a sign of barbarity. The Judeo-Christian ethic did not approve. Torture was left to "savages." One of the measures of civilization was the way man treated his fellow man. Provided, of course, that the fellow man was of the same color, race, religious persuasion, and ethnic stock. In the past fifty years or so, civilized man seems to have been slipping. More and more, the use of pain seems to have become organized, to be used by governments. The calculated use of pain seems to surround us, from the gangland "enforcer" to the armed forces.

Very little of the physical pain endured by the handicapped in our country is a result of deliberate cruelty. Occasionally, with the violence of the times, a handicapped person is physically set upon by moronic or sadistic people so doubtful of themselves that they try to bolster their sick egos by picking on someone ostensibly weaker. Children, who can be so kind and thoughtful, can also be amazingly cruel, but their cruelty to the handicapped is more apt to be verbal than physical, taking the form of taunts or imitation. Although sometimes the teasing that begins in fun can become cruel.

One of my children, a settled and good mother of several children today, had a streak of violence as a child, and shocked some people by her treatment of me at times. She loved me, as I loved her, and we both knew it. But sometimes, when some of her little friends were around, she would be very rough with me. It didn't bother me unduly because I knew what she was doing and why. She was saying, in her childish way, "Look, he can't walk very well, but he's strong and tough and I don't have to treat him with kid gloves." She didn't want anyone to feel sorry for her because she had a father who couldn't run with her or play some of the active games parents and children share; she wanted to show them they shouldn't be sorry for her and shouldn't be sorry for me, either. As long as I was seated, she would jump all over me, and not gently. But if I was standing, she was very careful not to bump into me, no matter how impulsively or blindly she seemed to be running.

When I was a child, other kids used to steal and hide my crutches occasionally, but this was just a form of teasing; they wouldn't ever hit me if I was standing up. I remember that one of my tentmates at a summer camp had one glass eye. He used to take out his false eye every night, and often in the morning it would have vanished. It would always show up in some unexpected place. Neither he nor his friends thought of this as cruel; it was simply a form of affectionate kidding that, in general, adults didn't understand. A child growing up with a physical handicap has enough real problems to lick without bothering about the teasing of his peers, which he is often pleased to see because it means that both he and his handicap have been accepted. I can remember playing inside one rainy day, and I asked for something, and one of my little friends said, "What's the matter, you crippled? Get it yourself." My mother, later, told me she had heard it and had been quite pleased to realize that was the way they treated me. My only worry had been that she might have been shocked—she thought they were such nice, polite children, she knew their parents. Even in families that communicate, there is (often amiable) misunderstanding between parents and children.

This form of teasing—name-calling, or stealing Pete's false eye—rarely caused physical pain, which was not its purpose. The mild mental discomfort it might cause was rarely serious or long lasting. It might even have been a form of bringing reality home to the one who was being teased. It might have been saying to him, "Look, you're our friend and we play with you, but there's one thing different about you. You know it, we know it, and it doesn't make any difference, but it's there."

Physical pain is something else again. It is debilitating. It has to be resisted and fought off, and this takes strength, mental and physical energy, which is one of the reasons that a continual or steady pain wears one down. It is not a matter of getting accustomed to it. The longer it lasts, the worse it gets. As I've said, I consider myself a coward because I hate and dread pain. I have a small, false reputation for bravery because I rarely make much of a fuss about it.

I have only found two nonmedical remedies for pain. One is distraction, the other is to analyze what's hurting you and why.

Distraction means, very simply, getting your mind on something else. It works pretty well on the smaller or shorter-term pains that bedevil us all from time to time. You can well ask, "How can I think about something else when I have a pain that is taking up all my attention?" That is why I said that fighting off pain takes energy. It takes energy because it requires concentration, focusing all your attention on something that is not your pain. That means a double concentration, concentrating on something and also concentrating against something.

The distraction technique works on a child, say, who is afraid of an injection he is about to get. You will often find a pediatrician or nurse administering a small, sharp slap to the fearful child's other hand or arm just before the injection is given. The child's brain indignantly takes in the unexpected slap and usually doesn't realize that while he was doing that, he has received the feared injection. Without a bit of advance preparation, the mind can handle only a certain amount of pain at any one time.

I've found radio or television a great help as a distraction, usually radio more than television. Television puts everything out for you; what you hear or see is quite evident. Radio

makes you use your mind a little more—you have to tell what
is going on from the sounds. On a TV mystery, for instance,
you see the door open and the villain enter. The same thing
on radio has to be conveyed by the sound of footsteps, of the
door opening and closing. It requires more attention or you
can't follow it, which makes it more useful as a distraction to
counter pain. I wouldn't think of going to a hospital as a
patient without a small transistor radio with an earphone so
I can listen without disturbing anyone else.

No form of distraction works as well for me as reading. But
then, I'm a reader by nature, and always have been. People
who use reading as an opiate often choose a type of book or
magazine that is unusual for them, an attention-grabber to
get their minds on something other than their troubles. That
is one reason why mysteries and light fiction are so popular
in hospitals.

When you go into a hospital for an operation, you know
before you go that it is going to be painful. You hope that the
pain will be minimized by the proper medication, but you
know that, no matter what efforts are made, there will be a
certain amount of pain, sometimes a good deal. When it is an
operation I know about in advance, not an emergency, I like
to look at an anatomy book or physiology book to find out
what they're trying to do and how they're planning to do it.
I also keep a little mental picture of the network of nerves
in the affected area. If I can mentally trace the pain from the
source, through the nerve system, up my spinal cord to the
brain, I feel better. If I can understand it, I feel somehow as
though I can control it.

A couple of years ago, I was rushed to the hospital in agony
for a cholecystectomy. For one thing, a bad gallbladder that
eventually ruptures is very painful. For another—I hadn't
prepared myself. If I could have told myself that this stupid

but sharp pain was simply caused by some gallstones blocking up some narrow ducts, I think I would have felt it less. But at first I didn't know what it was, only where it was. By the time they were able to operate and get rid of the trouble, it was simply a matter of recuperation, which I did surprisingly quickly. Surprising to the hospital, not to me—I expected it.

As must be obvious by now, I am a fatalist of sorts. But not a resigned fatalist. I feel that we can and must do everything within our power to control our own destinies. In the same way, I feel that up to a point we can control pain. It is a difficult thing to explain, but there comes a point, particularly when the pain is sudden and unexpected, when it gets inside of you. At that point, it controls you. There is also a point when you are battling it, if you win, when you get inside the pain. Which is the beginning of your control of the pain. As I said, it is difficult to explain, especially to one who hasn't experienced that feeling.

One of the safety valves people have is that they will faint, "pass out," when pain becomes too intense. I've had times when I hoped that I would lapse into unconsciousness, and other times, such as the occasion when I fell after I got out of my car and broke my hip, and tried to crawl back to the car, and kept passing out every time I moved a few inches. This annoyed me, as it delayed my inching progress. Just as I have never been able to pass out at will, in that case I wasn't able to remain conscious as long as I wanted, though I eventually made it back to the car.

Possibly because I've had some physical disabilities to contend with, I am a believer (limited) in mind over matter. For years, I've had a trick shoulder that dislocates on occasion. The first time it happened, I was in college, swinging down some narrow dormitory steps with a handrail on either side.

I was on my way to visit someone on the floor below and didn't want to spend time going to the elevator. I used to slide my crutches down the stairs and swing down on the handy railings. This time, one hand slipped, and I swung around in midflight, held by one hand, popping my right shoulder out of its socket. I was able to get it back after a while, but the muscles and tendons had been stretched, so the dislocation has recurred every now and then, usually when it hasn't happened for some time and I have grown careless. Once, reaching back to lock a rear door in a car, I dislocated my shoulder and couldn't get it back in place myself and had to go to a hospital to have it done. After that, I learned how to do it myself.

Because my legs aren't very good, I use my arms for many things and found this trick shoulder a great nuisance. There is an operation that can remedy this—athletes with easily dislocatable shoulders have it—but since my use of crutches means that I "walk on my arms," it would have incapacitated me for some time. I just learned to be careful and not let my right arm get into certain positions. For instance, I always put that arm into a jacket sleeve first, so I don't have to reach around with my right arm in back of me to put on a coat or jacket.

The problem with a dislocation of this type is that it hurts, and as long as you don't move, the pain subsides, only to return the moment you try to use it. It hurts quite a bit to try to get it back in place. The pain causes your muscles to tense, so that the knob at the top of your humerus has almost no chance of slipping easily back into its socket. When it does, it seems to do so with a crunch and a bang that momentarily nauseate you. Except for that one time I had to go to a hospital to have it done, I've always been able to do it myself, but it takes a bit of doing sometimes.

The trick is to force your muscles to relax and stay relaxed while they are hurting. They are crying out to be left alone and you are moving them, trying to get your shoulder back into its normal form. The work comes in making them stay relaxed while what you are doing to them hurts them more. The minute they tighten up, you might as well stop trying. And while you're trying to keep relaxed, you know that not only is moving them painful but that when the top of the humerus does slide in, it will momentarily hurt more and there will be a nerve "bang" not unlike the sensation of a dentist's drill striking a bad spot in a tooth.

For this purpose, I used to keep one small pure codeine pill with me, for use in case of emergency. If I couldn't get my shoulder back in place in a short time, I would swallow the pill, wait a few minutes for it to take effect, and then slide the arm back into place. Then I discovered that a quick shot of brandy or whiskey would work almost as well, so after using my last codeine pill, I didn't ask the doctor for any more.

Learning to relax a muscle isn't as hard as it may sound. I had to learn it when I was quite young, because I fell so often. As mentioned, I have had to learn to walk several times, and anyone who has watched a baby go through this process realizes that falling is a part of learning to walk. Performers are taught that the way to fall without injury is to relax when falling, which is contrary to instinct. Young babies fall relaxed, through inexperience, which is why they often fall from great heights without injury. As you get older, your instinct tells you to tighten the muscles before you hit, which usually causes more severe injuries. I had to learn to fall without trying to do any more than get particularly vulnerable parts out of the way. It's a little trick that has saved me a lot of trouble, even though I haven't always been able to use it.

As I've said, I have no good words to say for suffering. I think it should be avoided at all costs. But as we get older, we realize that we all have problems of one kind or another. A woman I know, a little younger than I, a bright, attractive divorcée who goes out with a number of men about her age, once said to me, "In a way, you're lucky. You had a basic physical problem early and you adjusted to it a long time ago. Now, in most ways, you're in better shape than most of the men I know."

I realize the truth of that statement whenever I attend a reunion of my college classmates or other alumni. At the time I attended college, I was one of the youngest in my class, due to my peculiar education. That little difference is unimportant now that my class has passed the fortieth anniversary of its graduation. When I see my contemporaries gathered together, I realize that I am physically lucky. Most of them seem to be taking pills for something, or they can't eat this or drink this, or they've become fanatics about the amount of sleep they must have or about heat or cold or drafts. This is not true of all of them, but of many. Some seem to be aging without worrying unduly about their health, but most seem to have specific physical problems to worry about. That is an unavoidable part of the aging process for most of us.

Many of my more or less healthy contemporaries awaken stiff or sore or coughing and bleary-eyed. They worry about smoking or not smoking, about drinking or not drinking, about cholesterol and butter and poly-unsaturated fats and salt-free foods. I listen to their complaints and sympathize and realize that, by and large, despite appearances, I'm healthy. And sometimes, listening, I'm amazed at the fact that they've lived so long with so little experience of more than minor, passing pains and disabilities. Many of them are realizing for the first time something I had to learn many years ago: there are some physical things they cannot do, and sometimes there will be pain. Some of these troubles are disappointments I am better able to handle than they, not because of anything superior in me but simply because they're not new to me; I'm accustomed to them. And, at an age when there are apt to be aches and pains, few have learned my simple lesson. I suppose that could be called the silver-lining department, but seeing your friends and peers experiencing troubles you might be better able to handle is not a pleasure.

The lesson I had to learn and can't explain to them is that pain is largely in the mind. I don't mean it's imaginary. It's like that tree, silent or noisy, falling in the deserted forest. There is no pain until the brain receives and translates the message. And pain can be lessened by concentrating on ignoring it and thinking of something else.

I'm talking about the kind of pain that most of us are apt to experience, not about torture or deliberate pain. I have no idea how I would stand up to that, and I don't want to find out. My guess is not well, because I would probably be angry and lose any detachment that might enable me to withstand it—my brain would not be in control. I don't think that anyone who has not been tortured has a right to pass judgment on the actions of those who have, whether the torture was physical punishment or imprisonment or confinement or interrogation. I can understand the reaction of the late Admiral Parsons (then Captain), a brave and intelligent man, who borrowed a handgun to carry in his pocket before setting out in the *Enola Gay* for Hiroshima. The only man on the mission who knew the workings of the atomic bomb, he didn't want to have to trust to his courage if he should be captured.

But most ordinary, run-of-the-mill pains can be controlled by the mind. An ordinary, run-of-the-mill pain is one being felt by someone else. A mildly cheerful thing to remember is that the worst pains are ones we don't feel but anticipate. Which is how I know I'm a coward—I have a good, active imagination. One of the ways civilization has progressed has been in the elimination or reduction of pain. Many pains that were once expected to be borne stoically as a part of life are now considered unnecessary.

Pain, as I have said, is purely subjective. I can only talk about it as I know it, and the theories expressed are my own. I have talked about this subject with a good many people who have had similar experiences. I have not found many areas of agreement. Some people have told me that my method of knowing what was being done wouldn't work for them— they didn't want to know anything about it. Two men considered the idea of watching an operation being performed on them as morbid. Many considered my idea of concentrating on something else ridiculous, but one man said he'd gotten through one bad siege by trying to remember the most pleasant sexual experiences he'd ever had. Many agreed that the worry and fear of an anticipated pain were usually worse than the actuality.

As the study of medicine has continued, more and more has been learned about the human body and its nervous system, and more has been learned about making pain bearable by keeping knowledge of it from reaching the brain. It wasn't so long ago that operations were conducted without anesthetics or with only the crudest forms. Sufferers were given rags to stifle their screams or moans, or a bullet or piece of wood on which to bite. Anesthetics have not only improved in quality but have been more localized, so they can block off the pain in one section or area. So, today, if you have to have a tooth pulled or a bone broken or an offending organ cut open or excised, be glad it is being done to you now when so many pain-killers are available and their use is considered routine.

CHAPTER SEVEN

Other Members
of
the Family

The family of a handicapped person is extremely important to him, and to his development if he is a child. And having someone in the family with a handicap affects the others in many ways. The family question has to be looked at from both points of view. A British doctor, Mary Sheridan, wrote in *The Handicapped Child and His Home* (London, 1965) that it is no exaggeration to say: "In the background of every individual handicapped child there is always a handicapped family."

As usual, I have to use myself and my immediate family as prime examples, because these are the people I know best and watched and listened to longest. No matter how friendly you may be with another family, it is impossible for an outsider to know its inner tensions, despairs, and gratifications. It's easy enough to misjudge one's own family. As I have said,

I was fortunate in many ways, and one of the most important was to have been born into a close-knit, affectionate, intelligent and articulate family. My immediate relatives consisted of a mother and a father, a sister a couple of years older than I, and, later, a younger brother. In addition, as far as closeness was concerned, there were grandparents and their children, which meant uncles, aunts, and cousins, though not sufficiently numerous to be reckoned by the dozens.

I have mentioned my parents enough, but they will come back into the story at times. My sister is another matter. Unlike many siblings, we always got along well. When we were quite young, we worked out a way to drive our parents crazy, something at which all children seem to be adept. I don't think we ever talked about it and came up with a plan, we just did it. If she was punished, with or without justice (in our minds), she would bear up stoically under the punishment, and I would put up a fuss, even crying noisily if necessary. If I was punished, she would fuss and cry. This was not pure unselfishness: we knew it put our parents on the spot and had a tendency to lessen the punishment. We used the technique until we grew too old to make it effective. Our little brother was so much a junior, ten years younger than my sister, that he was never a part of that club.

My sister's name was Jeanne, a pretty name that caused her trouble all her early life because it was pronounced in the French manner. At school, others would tease her by calling her John and saying it was a boy's name. As I said, we got along very well together and we still do. But as I grew older and looked more closely into people instead of just accepting them without thinking, I was never able to understand why she didn't hate me. She was the first, the oldest, and a girl. All of a sudden, she had a rival in the family, which is normal enough. But then I came down with polio, turning the house upside down, and unavoidably receiving the bulk of our parents' attention, and that of strangers and friends. When I grew old enough to think about it and ask her if she hated me, she answered no, it hadn't occurred to her. The only reason I can see is that she was, and is, one of the naturally good people.

I do not come from a violent family. My mother has a temper and is quite volatile, one of those people who can blow up quickly and unpredictably and get over it just as quickly, with no holdovers. Her temper was always expressed vocally, never physically. My father, a much quieter person, had a temper that he didn't like to show and usually kept under tight control. My sister, brother, and I shared a certain gentleness that I later decided came from growing up with love.

My mother and father were totally different, in appearance and temperament. My mother was tall, quick, imperious, talkative, brilliant, and changeable. My father was short, broad, thorough, stubborn, quiet, and stable. They used to fight at times. As children, we watched and listened to these verbal and temperamental fusses without alarm, more with a sense of condescending amusement. We were not upset because we knew, with the wisdom of children, that they were just letting off steam and there was no lack of love behind it. I can remember my father getting furious, turning livid but not raising his voice, picking up his hat and cane and storming out of the house. He would start to slam the front door in his fury and stop it before it could slam shut and make a noise. In fifteen minutes or an hour or two, he would come back, having walked off his anger, ashamed of himself for having been angry, and pleased that he hadn't shown it.

My mother was the volatile, noticeable one, but my father was what held her together. I always had the notion that she was sort of a ball, a bubble flying off in all directions but never going too far because she was somehow tethered to my father, circling around him. He was her center of gravity. It was an unlikely marriage to look at, but it worked because, no matter how much they might annoy one another, each had a good deal of respect and admiration for the other. My mother was an early feminist—a suffragette, as they used to be called—and a pacifist at a time when that wasn't popular or fashionable, but my father backed her all the way. It wasn't until I was a good deal older that I realized how lucky we had been to grow up in a home where we knew there was love. There are dozens of family stories to show this mutual respect, but they don't really belong in a story about the handicapped. Except that trying to bring up a family in which one of the boys could walk only with extreme difficulty must have presented unusual problems.

Then there were my mother's parents, both of them characters. My grandfather, a large and strikingly handsome man, was a very successful portrait photographer, an artist who made more money than he could spend, and he tried all ways. He was an elemental force in a way, of a type that no longer exists, a cultivated city man but still a sort of frontier Westerner. He believed that he had not only the right but the duty to say what he thought without necessarily lowering his voice. He never wanted to hurt anyone, but he wanted to make sure that his point of view was unmistakably on record. He cannot have been the easiest man in the world to be married to, but he was a wonderful person for a little boy to call Grandpa.

His type of individualism was a product of the time, the place, and his own temperament. He liked to drink, and, in a gentlemanly way, he ate and drank himself to death. He was in a position to do what he wanted to do, and he wanted

to do things in his own way. His office was his studio, a building he had had constructed in the form of a French chateau,
including a large tower. This meant that on every floor above
the first there was a large, round tower room. The studio was
a wonderful place to play in bad weather, filled with works
of art, suits of armor, swords, halberds, old rifles on the wall,
and trunks and sea chests under the round windows,
crammed with things to play with for hours, like bundles of
Confederate money.

He knew everyone and everyone knew him. He had been
decorated by many foreign governments, but the only deco-
ration he seemed to value was that of the Académie Fran-
çaise. And even in this, I heard (because this was long before
I was born), he had to show his independence. He was supposed to go to Paris to be honored, but reportedly said, "If
they want to give me something, let them come here and
give it to me." So they did.

He loved his horses, but was an early automobile fancier,
and reportedly had the first Cadillac in the city and then the
first eight-cylinder one, later switching unexpectedly to a
competitor, the now forgotten Peerless. He was one of the
world's worst drivers, which I knew even as a child. I didn't
realize until I had children of my own how much of a strain
that must have put on my parents.

Because every Saturday afternoon he would pick me up
and I'd go to his house for dinner and to spend the night, I
always had my own room at my grandparents' place. When
I think back to the meals that were served there, it's a wonder to me that any of the family lived to an old age. A standard, no-occasion, family dinner was at least five or six courses,
with appropriate wines. Grandpa lived well and enjoyed it.
He also had a thing about paying rent, and wouldn't live in
any building he didn't own. His house, only a few minutes'

walk from the studio, was huge in an old-fashioned way. It included a stable—later half-turned into a garage, with its own gasoline pump, as was customary at the time—a tennis court, and a summerhouse, vined and latticed and paved with beer bottles set upside down in the earth or concrete.

On Sunday morning, Grandpa would wake me by throwing the funny papers at me and I'd join him for a big breakfast. Then we'd go for a drive. Driving with Grandpa was an experience. He was polite and gracious, but not behind the wheel. Traffic laws were for other people. There were one or two areas for speeding, and Grandpa always had a big, fast car. Once every so often, a motorcycle would come up behind us, signaling with its siren. The policeman would pull up next to the driver, looking to see who was driving so fast, and would pull away, smiling and waving as he drove on, mouthing a greeting. This should have given me no respect for the law, but I never had any idea that I rated that kind of treatment. I've been driving for years and have never had a ticket for speeding or any moving violation.

Grandpa would have been very impatient at stoplights today, but there were very few of them at the time. However, there were corners with traffic policemen, and if Grandpa was held up for what he thought was an unconscionable time, he would honk his horn to get the policeman's attention, and eventually go through the same procedure as with the speed cop—starting with a glare and ending with a smile and a wave.

Those Sunday drives were something to remember. Grandpa was a fascinating conversationalist, and few people had him alone as much as I did. No matter how fast he wanted to drive, our progress would often be slow because everyone recognized him. He'd have to stop to talk to too many people—sometimes the Mayor, or one particular

United States Senator who seemed to cherish him, or a gardener. I found out years later that Grandpa had stayed up a whole night with the Senator, who was bent, for some reason, on committing suicide. Usually, a child going places with an adult who stops to talk to people finds it dull. I rarely did, because the people were interesting and unexpected things happened.

One incident seemed right out of a book. We were stopped at a corner for a conversation with a man who had hailed us, a middle-aged man and a dull conversationalist. When the man turned to go, Grandpa apologized to me for the delay, and asked, "You know who that is?" I said no, and Grandpa told me his name, one of the most prominent businessmen in the city and a leading, conservative Republican. Grandpa, a small- and large-"D" Democrat, said, "I'm sorry he was so long-winded, but I couldn't stop him. He's the meanest son of a bitch in town."

Grandpa did not say things like that sotto voce. The man hadn't gone far and he turned back toward the car, his tight features beginning to turn red. "What did you call me?" he asked.

"You heard me," Grandpa said. "I said you were the meanest son of a bitch in the city. And you are, you know."

Those were fighting words at the time. The man knew it, Grandpa knew it, even I knew it.

My grandfather was, in his own individualistic way, a fancy dresser. He would have called anyone else who dressed that way a dude. He wore huge, flowing ties and smart hats and carried a pencil-thin cane. When driving, he wore soft, yellow, skin-tight gloves. While his opponent fumed outside the car, making the motions of a man loosening his coat, Grandpa, slowly and meticulously, began peeling off his fancy gloves.

I sat there, overcome with fear and anxiety. Fear that they would fight and fear that they wouldn't. I wasn't anxious about the outcome. Although my grandfather was a few years older, he was also larger, over six feet tall, and he still played tennis whenever he could.

Nothing happened. The angry man outside the car said something like "Hmph," and walked away. Grandpa started putting his gloves back on, and I started to relax. Until Grandpa said, "Mean. And yellow, too." Not very dignified behavior for two men who were powers in the community, but they have to be seen in the context of their times.

I suppose, in a way, I was a favorite of my grandfather's. Parents and grandparents are not supposed to have favorites, but they do, whether or not they will admit it or show it. Grandpa moved in a world of artists, but he was an intensely physical man. I don't think I was favored because I couldn't walk, but perhaps I was because he had to show me he didn't hold it against me. And he was proud of me, as grandparents are apt to be, because he thought I was bright.

The fact that I didn't start RCA shows that I wasn't as bright as a proud grandfather might think. In the early days of radio, sets were large, unreliable, and expensive. I started building them, as boys did in those days when a good radio cost several hundred dollars but you could build one for much less, and often a better one. Interested people bought the latest magazines about them, as new circuits were coming out month after month, each one supposedly better than its predecessor. I had started with a crystal detector, earphones, and a pair of honeycomb coils for tuning, and eventually graduated to vacuum tubes and a loudspeaker of sorts. I remember the acid from a storage battery, and my carelessness with it, ate a hole through a portion of a large Oriental rug in my room, annoying my mother no end.

Grandpa once asked me if I could make him a radio that would work better than the one he had, and I said yes without hesitation. We settled for my estimate of $75 without a speaker. I built it, and he came by one evening to pick it up and me. Some of his friends were at his house and he proudly showed us off, his grandson, whom they knew, and the new toy I'd built him. Was it a flop? Anything connected with Grandpa would have to be a real flop or a rousing success, which is what the new radio was. For no reason at all, after showing how it would get KSD, the local station, and KDKA in Pittsburgh, I started dial-hopping, and picked up the station in Jefferson City, the state capital. Someone was making a speech about, of all people, my grandfather, who was very much against Prohibition, both personally and in principle. As was the case with most of his views, he made no secret of his feelings. Someone in Jefferson City was attacking Grandpa's views on the subject.

There could hardly have been a more auspicious debut for a new radio set. I had orders for three or four other sets from Grandpa's friends that evening. Why, after that fine start, I didn't go into the manufacture of radios, I don't know. But after I filled those orders, I stopped building them, except for myself. The circuits were becoming standardized, mass production was setting in, and it was becoming possible to buy sets that were better than I could make, and for less money.

It's impossible at this late date for me to figure out whether I would have been as close to my grandfather if I had not had polio. I don't think it made any difference. But because he was who and what he was, my life was more pleasant and interesting than it would have been otherwise. Somewhere, there is a picture of me as a little boy standing next to a tall, good-looking, smiling man who has his hand on my shoulder. The man signed the picture, too, with something like, "For

Joe, with Best Wishes . . . George Sisler." Sisler was the no-longer-existing St. Louis Browns' version of Mickey Mantle or Willie Mays. He was a polite, soft-spoken man, a future Hall of Famer, a college graduate and a gentleman in a period when many ballplayers were roughnecks. It was a nice picture to keep in my room for other boys to see. It showed the only time I ever met him, a gift from Grandpa.

As was my first flight in a plane, when I was eleven or twelve. Some kind of air show was being held in St. Louis, and Grandpa, who was interested in all things new and different, took me to the field a day or two before the show was officially opened. I was taken up by then Lieutenant Al Williams, the speed-record holder. After which, Grandpa began to worry about his daughter's reaction to the news, and made me promise not to say anything about it, a promise I kept for many years. Grandpa couldn't roughhouse with me or teach me how to behave on horseback as he had his own children, but he got some pleasure out of me, as I did from him. I don't know what my parents ever said to him, if anything, about how I should be treated, but I know his wife, my grandmother, must have been a different problem.

How do you convince a grandmother that rushing over to comfort and pick up a fallen grandson is the wrong tactic? I know that I fell often for many years, and my grandmother never came from wherever she was to help me up. Nor did anyone in her house. I still remember that there would be a crash and down I'd go, and my grandmother's cheery voice would follow from somewhere: "You dropped something."

Whether she thought of this as a way to let me know that she knew I had fallen, or whether my parents or someone else thought of it, I'll never know. But knowing the way grandparents generally feel and react, I realize it must have been quite a job to persuade her that the thing to do was stay away instead of picking me up. I was spoiled in other ways, which is a special privilege granted to grandparents. I had the habit even then of reading to music. I would sit in a huge club chair, select the records I wanted to hear, and start to work my way through the reading material I had put within arm's reach. The chauffeur or yard man would rewind the stand-up Victrola and change the records, while I sat and read and nibbled at cookies from the jar next to the books. It was my idea of heaven for a few hours at a certain age, and in my memory is somehow mixed in with that cheery "You dropped something."

I always loved and admired my grandmother, but I didn't realize how much of a person she was until I was almost grown. She had been born in St. Louis at about the time Fort Sumter was fired upon, and I always thought of her as a lovely hothouse flower, a spoiled daughter and wife in a simpler era of large houses, formal entertaining, and plenty of servants. She had been known as a beauty and retained much of her looks and fine complexion almost until she died in her nineties. She said she never used soap and water on her hands and face, only cold cream. When she was in her seventies or older, she had some kind of intestinal stoppage and couldn't take any food. She was put in the hospital, where she kept telling her doctors that all she needed was some champagne. Finally, they gave her some. What do you do with an old lady who has always behaved as though she were a duchess and has been treated like one? A couple of days later, she was home again, good for a few more decades.

As a child, I saw her as a woman who ran a big house, but I thought everything was done for her. I can't recall ever seeing her cook anything more complicated than a piece of toast. Many years later, when she lived as a widow in an apartment hotel with her old chauffeur taking care of her, I suddenly realized that the food she served there was about the same as when she'd had a large house. Of course, if it was a large gathering, everyone would go downstairs to eat in the hotel dining room. Finally, she didn't have the car any more. She didn't go out much, but she still had the chauffeur. He'd been with her for years, and, as she said, she was used to him and, besides, what could he do, where could he get a job at his age?

It wasn't until I was half grown that I realized there was a good deal more to her than the helpless, charming person she seemed to be. I knew she had run a large, active household, had brought up four children (another daughter died in her pre-teens), and had held to her own identity in a family of strong characters. At a period when people, particularly women, were supposed to age quietly and gracefully, she had stayed young. She had a strong time sense, despite the custom of being fashionably late. I knew that if I was to pick her up at noon, I could get to her place at 11:55 and find her standing outside, asking where I'd been. And if she was taking a trip, she liked to be at the station an hour before the train was supposed to leave—as though the train would dare leave without her!

One day, when she was about eighty-five, she went downtown to do some shopping, wearing her usual high-heeled shoes. A spike heel caught in a hole just inside a store entrance, put there to catch a stay to hold a door open in certain weather, and she fell and broke her hip. She never walked again. A decade or two earlier, it might have been fatal because the aged died of broken hips, due to various diseases and impairments developed by internal organs because of lack of exercise. By the time she broke her hip, the medical profession had discovered the virtues of penicillin and movement, so she lived for almost another decade.

It was a family custom to go to her home for Sunday dinner, as it had been with a smaller family and a large house. By this time, I was living in New York, with children of my own. One Sunday when I had flown in the night before, I went early to have a chance to talk to Grandma before my mother and my sister and her husband and their three boys arrived. But I found her too busy to have much time for talk. She was reading every word of the sport sections of the two Sunday papers. I said I was surprised, I didn't think she was that interested in sports.

She looked around to make sure that no one else had come in with me. "I'm not," she said. "But my three great-grandsons are. And they'll be here in an hour, so I have to read every word of the sport pages so I can listen to them and ask questions as though I know what I'm talking about. I have to read them slowly and carefully so I can memorize some of the names and figures of what happened yesterday."

It made me realize why going to Grandma's—or Great-Grandma's, or Mother's, as the case might be—for Sunday dinner wasn't a duty but a pleasure. You could look forward to your favorite foods being served—you'd expect that from any grandparent raised as she had been—but also she worked to keep up with young people's interests, be they sports or current songs or books or art. Because she was that kind of a person, she kept young, and young people around her.

I remember getting a letter from Grandma early in January after hearing my friends complain about a dull New Year's Eve party because, they said, we were too old. Grandma had written, "Had the most wonderful New Year's Eve. So many people came in. Had nothing to drink but champagne"—there she was, on a champagne kick again—"and about two in the morning started playing cards and won $40 at poker." As I've said, I had built up a dislike of what

I called old ladies, but I never considered my grandmother one, and I don't think she thought of herself that way either. If she had, would she have bought a Braille machine, after she broke her hip and couldn't get around much, learned to use it, and spent her spare time translating things into Braille so the blind could read them?

My mother and father, my sister, and my grandparents each had his or her own problems connected with living with me and learning how to treat me when I was growing up with a handicap. My brother, Dickie, had a different problem. He was eight years younger than I, and by the time he was aware and growing, I'd had my illness and many operations and was pretty well set in a pattern of life that included a physical handicap. What effect does this have on a kid brother? I don't know. He had problems that weren't the same as mine, problems that had nothing to do with physical abilities or lack of them. As with all kid brothers, there were times when he was a nuisance, just as I had been to my sister at times. But he was a wonderful kid. I don't say that now because he was killed; I thought it and said it at the time.

I've said I never understood why my sister didn't and doesn't hate me; as far as I know, Dickie had no reason to hate me, and didn't. Our growing-up experiences were completely different. By the time he was in high school, the stock market had crashed, we had moved to southern Illinois, and life had changed for the nation and for us. He had to adjust to living in a small town where our family had no roots but a certain automatic acceptance, as well as a mild resentment because we owned a factory, by that time the only large employer in the Depression-hit town. And he had to adjust to the usual problems of adolescence, which included the fact that he was shooting up like a stalk of the local corn. He had been a thin, blond, medium-sized boy, but suddenly he started to grow every time you took your eyes off of him for a moment. It didn't go on forever, of course; he leveled off at six feet three or four, with legs that had to be tucked in whenever he sat down.

World War II was brewing in Europe by the time he went away to college, first to Antioch and then to the University of Wisconsin. He knew he would be in the war, and wanted to be in it as a flyer, so he started taking courses to learn to fly. He tried to enlist in the Air Corps, but it kept turning him down because he was too thin for his height, so he went on a doctor's diet to gain weight, and kept on taking more flying courses. Eventually, there weren't any more civilian courses he could take; he was rated an instructor in cross-country flying, as I remember, and though he hadn't gained a pound, the Air Corps accepted him, as he had thought it would. He was one of two men without previous airline-pilot ratings who were accepted into a special group of experienced flyers for a shortened, intensive training period. He was reportedly the last trainee of his height put into a fighter plane as a pilot, but he was evidently pretty good, as he ended up flying as a test or check pilot in all kinds of experimental craft. He was enjoying himself. He liked flying and he had found something at which he excelled.

My upset at his death was mitigated to a certain extent by the fact that he died doing the thing he wanted to do. I never talked to him about the effect my disability might have had on him. I might have afterward, but there was never a chance. I think my learning to fly was partly because he was so much in favor of it. He had an idea that after the war a lot of the trainers being built for the Air Corps could be bought cheaply by the civilian population and the two of us could get one and have fun with it. He used to phone me and talk about it, and the only time I can remember my handicap ever being mentioned was when he was enthusiastically talking about a specific plane, and he said it was so easy to get in and out of. He was killed before he reached twenty-five, so I don't know what his considered opinion would have been of the effect of having an older brother with a physical handicap.

The importance of the way the other members of a family treat a handicapped child is hard to overemphasize. Outsiders, friends coming into contact with the family, will usually pattern their treatment of a handicapped child on the treatment they see the family give him. This is either an unconscious reaction, or they figure that the way his mother, father, or brothers treat him must be the right way.

One of the major problems a handicapped person has to face is how he relates to others, and the way he handles personal relationships is often based on his place as an individual in the family. If he is ignored, he may feel himself worthless, something very easy for the handicapped to do. If he is treated with too much kindness, he may grow to expect the same consideration from others, and become resentful when the world doesn't treat him that way. If he is accepted as just another member of the family with his individual quirks and foibles, outsiders, seeing this, are apt to treat him the same way, which can make for a healthy give-and-take when he is not dealing with people who are related to him and know him well.

I had the usual number of relatives, and my family, which was sociable, had a large number of friends, so there were a lot of people who saw me in my home environment and took their cues from that. There were others, distant relatives and not-so-close friends, who wanted to feel sorry for me, but their attitude meant no more to me than that of strangers who could be forgiven because they didn't know any better. A good deal of the progress a handicapped person makes toward leading a normal life depends on how he feels about himself as a person, and much of that is shaped by how his family feels about him and treats him. Love and kindness help in any situation, but without intelligent thought, they are not enough to make a handicapped child into a person.

At some point, when I was quite young, I had a small household chore: I had to answer the telephone if no one else was near enough to pick it up automatically. We lived in a large house with enough help to handle the phone, but this was a deliberate move on the part of my parents to give me some small, daily, household responsibility. At the time, I didn't get around very well. If I was sitting down when the phone rang, it meant I had to get my crutches, get up, and then lock my braces and walk to the telephone. That took some time, and the phone would keep ringing. Some of my parents' friends thought this was cruel, but it was explained to them that most young boys have certain minor chores, even if it's only running to the corner for a paper or cigarettes. I heard some of the arguments, and I have to say I never resented having to answer the phone, though if none of the adults was home there were times I would call to a maid to pick up the phone, and sometimes she would and sometimes not. Or sometimes answering, "All right, I will this time, but if your parents catch me doing it I'll be shot and it'll be your fault."

Obviously, my family's attitude toward my physical problems helped steer me in the direction I took. My illness must have been a terrific blow to my parents, something totally unexpected that had to change their lives. It must have been very hard on my mother, in particular, as most of the day-to-day work on me fell to her because she was at home all day. My father was downtown most of the day. Besides, he was a man, accustomed to responsibility and about a decade older than my mother, who had spent her early years being a bright, beautiful, spoiled daughter and then a spoiled wife.

Then suddenly, before she was thirty, she had to face a grim reality: a child who might not live and, if he did, would never be quite the same as other children. As good people do, when she met a big enough challenge, she faced up to it. Despite this, she has remained spoiled, first as a child and wife, then as a mother, now as a spoiled grandmother and great-grandmother. She had to have the courage of her convictions, at a time when the treatment of handicapped children was far different from today's. It must have been difficult to stand up to her friends who thought she was cruel making me answer the phone, who thought she was foolish to let me have a car and drive it to the East Coast and back every time I went to college and returned home, who thought she was wrong to encourage my interest in sports in which I'd never be able to participate on an equal footing if at all.

Fortunately, for many years she had the help and backing of a man who thought she was right in what she did. I'm not trying to take any credit away from my father—he had the solid, steadfast character she needed to keep her going along the way she thought right—but he was the first to admit that she set the pace and made the major decisions in how my illness was to be handled.

And what reward does she get for it? In public, I say she's spoiled. I'm not saying anything behind her back that I haven't said to her face; she acknowledges it and says she likes being spoiled. I've also told her she spent many years of hard work trying to make me independent and now regrets her success, to which she says she doesn't regret it at all—but won't I listen to her some time about something?

CHAPTER EIGHT

Transportation

When you can't walk, transportation is a major issue. That would seem to be self-evident but might need a little elaboration which gets back to basics. Anyone with a physical handicap of any kind tends to use whatever substitute he can to make up for it. A person who is physically mute will try to acquire and perfect himself in other means of communication so as not to be shut off from others. When mobility is your problem, an artificial means to help you get about is of paramount importance. It gets to the whole point of rehabilitation, which is any means of enabling a handicapped person to lead a useful life.

A person with a handicap is different from one without it. Efforts—his own and those of others—to enable him to lead a useful life have to be based on eliminating or reducing the difference. A skeletal-motor handicap brings in the basic difficulty of locomotion. If I place what may seem an inordinate amount of importance on the handicapped's use of the automobile, for instance, it is because I do not think it is inordinate. People have been crippled since the beginning of time, by wars, accidents, birth defects or injuries, and disease. People moved by their own feet or those of others, and later by horse. If they moved in any other way—by water, for instance—they had to get to the boat or raft somehow.

I've known and talked to myriads of the handicapped, and the number who are comfortable with or can handle horses is microscopic. And until this century, getting around depended largely on horses, or a horse. This severely limited the activities of the handicapped. For many of them the development of the automobile was of primary importance, although few realized it at the time. It gave the handicapped one of the things they needed most, independence of transportation. This is something most people take for granted from the time they start walking. People take their physical blessings as a matter of course until these are removed or impaired. I don't think that anyone who has always been able to move about as he wished can realize how important that simple, basic faculty is. I don't think that anyone without a mobility handicap can realize what the automobile has meant to people with motor handicaps.

Fortunately for me, my parents realized this early. They had promised me my own car as soon as I was legally old enough to drive, which was sixteen at the time. Missouri hadn't thought about drivers' licenses so early in powered transportation's history. Automobiles were more primitive then, without power assists or automatic transmissions, which made driving more of a physical problem. By the time I reached my sixteenth birthday, I was driving our car with no trouble, having worked out my own system.

For the benefit of those who weren't around in those early years, a car was a much simpler mechanism then than it is now, and driving was more complicated. The self-starter had been invented and was in general use, but all cars had cranks, too, and I learned how to crank a car. There was a mystique about cranking, as there was about double-clutching, which a later generation took to sports cars and "four on the floor" rediscovered. As for cranking, all you had to have was a little knowledge about what to do and some arm muscles, which I had. You were always cautioned about doing it wrong and ending up with a broken arm. That was a subject of cartoons and supposedly a common occurrence that I heard of often but never saw happen.

The automatic choke was not yet in use, nor the automatic spark timing control, so cars had more manual controls. There were the clutch and the usual foot brake and hand brake (today's parking brake, then called the emergency brake), and the foot throttle, or accelerator. On the dashboard was the choke, for use when starting. On the steering wheel were a hand throttle and a hand spark control, for use when cranking or starting the engine, to be retarded when starting and advanced to its proper setting as soon as the engine was running. By the time I was driving, the hand windshield wiper had been replaced by an automatic one, operated by a vacuum on the intake manifold. If you were fancy, you had two windshield wipers, one on the driver's side and another on the righthand side.

In those days, long before automatic transmissions or even synchro-mesh transmissions, shifting gears was a fine art. With only one foot and leg that worked, I had to devise a system of starting, shifting, and stopping, which I did. It needed a feeling and an ear for things mechanical, which I had. I eventually got the system down to a point where I used the clutch only to start from a complete standstill. I would use my good right foot on the clutch and a hand on the hand throttle and put the car into the lowest gear and accelerate. I taught myself to shift from first to second and second to third without the clutch, by getting the engine speed to coincide with the gear speed. When coming to a complete stop, there was always one point where the axle speed and engine speed were the same, at which point I would slide the gearshift lever into neutral. It sounds more complicated than it was, and is more difficult to describe than it is to do, because it became second nature to me.

Many years later, after driving with automatic transmissions for a couple of decades, I rented a car in Europe. At that time, almost all the rental cars outside the United States, whether American-made or foreign, had manually operated transmissions, either stick shifts on the floor or hand shifts on the steering column. Of course, the hand-operated spark control and accelerator on the steering wheel had disappeared along with the open road. I rented a medium-sized European car, and two minutes after taking it, I opened the hood and set up the idling speed so I'd be able to start from a dead stop even on a slight hill. I drove the little car through Western Europe from the Baltic to the Mediterranean, through the flatlands of Jutland to the mountains of Italy, Spain, and Switzerland, with no trouble at all. I was pleased to discover that my driving system, developed by desire and necessity so many years earlier, came back and seemed as natural as it had when I was in college.

Taking that gearshift car in Europe wasn't as rash as it sounds. I had done it a couple of years earlier in Puerto Rico, where I had rented a non-automatic Chevrolet after driving a Volkswagen for a couple of hours and finding it uncomfortable and difficult for me to drive. And on an earlier trip to

Europe, I had rented a large American convertible with an automatic transmission for a couple of weeks on the Riviera. The only trouble with that was the car was too wide for exploring properly some of the small towns in France and Italy; with those wide fenders you had to be very careful not to brush pedestrians off the sidewalks.

Mobility, as I pointed out, has been extremely important to me. As a child, the Irish Mail described earlier enabled me to keep up with the other children, after a fashion; then the family car, driven by my mother or the chauffeur, enabled me to get around, or be taken around. Then, as soon as it was legal, I was driving myself. As I've grown older, I have discovered that stairs and bad weather are more troublesome to me than they were earlier. Either they're more of a problem physically, or I've grown more cautious and less foolhardy with advancing age.

I don't like wet weather, but it doesn't bother me unduly unless it is cold enough to cause freezing. One of my peculiarities, which probably has nothing to do with any physical infirmity, is the fact that I'm usually too hot and never wear a hat or overcoat. I don't mind cold as long as it isn't too slippery underfoot. I think that one reason I don't wear a hat or own an umbrella is that they're difficult to handle, particularly in a wind, when both hands are busy with crutches.

Ice, of course, isn't the only cause of slippery terrain. I've been in parts of Latin America where beautiful tile is used on the sidewalks, and during and after a tropical shower they become as slick as a skating rink. And in some lovely but remote areas of Yucatán, even steppingstones, put there to keep you from sinking into the mud, get coated with moss and slime that make your crutches slide as though they've been greased.

I learned quite young that there were certain things I could do and certain things I couldn't handle easily or safely. Years before everyone else used them, I had snow tires on my car in the winter. I figured if it was bad enough so that cars would have trouble starting, stopping, or climbing hills, it would be worse for me on foot. I also wasn't very useful carrying things. The weight wasn't as much of a problem for me as the bulk. Today, the popular shopping bags with handles make carrying many things easy for me, and I usually keep a spare one in the car trunk and another on the back seat. Certain things, not necessarily large or heavy, are difficult to hold while also maneuvering a crutch. I have worn out more briefcases than I can remember, and a large amount of luggage that is not rectangular.

A suitcase of the usual shape has a handle in the middle, which makes it difficult to grasp while one hand is holding a crutch handle, but a wedge-shaped case like the old Boston bags, or Gladstones, can be carried without too much trouble. I have also accumulated a collection of airline flight bags because they are shaped so they can be carried easily while one hand is guiding a crutch. I have them in at least five different sizes, the largest being one from an airline I neither like nor use, but which had the largest bag of its type I've seen. When I travel by car, I may put in the trunk a large rectangular bag with an extra pair of shoes, two suits and other necessities in it, and also have in the trunk an airline bag with enough clothes and toiletries to hold me for several days and overnight stops.

For many years, I have traveled almost exclusively by car or plane. Ships are lovely, if you can find one going where you want to go, but they are not for me. Gangplanks are not easy to walk on and are apt to be steeply angled, depending on the tide. Even the largest ocean liners, the floating hotels, are not always steady, and are built with high dividers to step over, not to keep me out but to keep out the waters. I stopped using trains long before most of the American traveling public gave up on them, though when I was young I used to enjoy being on a crack train for a long journey, and all my youthful trips between St. Louis and Boston were by train. How else could you do it in those days? As most travelers know, European railways, with government ownership or backing, have not been allowed to deteriorate the way the once wonderful American rail system has. But, for the handicapped, the problem of getting on and off remains, as well as certain difficulties that have to do with walking on a moving train.

In New York City and most of its commuter stations, the platforms have been built so that they're level with the car exits and entrances so one doesn't have to clamber aboard via a couple of steep, difficult steps. The only train that I take willingly in the United States now is the Metroliner between New York and Washington. In all the New York stations, the platform matches the height of the car floor, and at the Washington station, the two end tracks set aside for Metroliner use have raised platforms, the only tracks in the terminal with such an arrangement.

The good trains in Europe today seem like the "good old days" of American railroading as far as comfort, service, and convenience are concerned, once you're aboard. But their platforms seem even lower than ours, and the steps in the cars even steeper.

One fall, when I expected to go to several places in Europe and be there for some little time, I bought one of those handy Eurailpasses that let you go first-class on any European railway, prepaid. I enjoyed it very much, and flew or drove only for short trips, and rented a car if I expected to stay in one area for a long time. For anyone who likes to travel as much as I do, just having a usable Eurailpass in your pocket gives you a pleasant feeling. But the difficulty of getting on and off the trains has made me hesitant about doing it again.

Airplanes and airports are often planned in a way that makes it difficult for anyone with a mobility handicap to travel. In many places, you arrive on a plane, have to climb down the loading stairs to reach the ground, and then climb up and down other flights of stairs inside the airport building to get to your luggage or taxi or both. But in almost all airports there is another way to do it: if you ask, you will find that somewhere there is an elevator or an inclined ramp, not necessarily put there for you, but to allow baggage to be wheeled in and out, or off and on. Most major airports today have those handy "jetways," the ingenious telescoping tubes that allow passengers to step from the plane door into the airport building on the same level. The nicest airport in this respect is also the country's safest, according to many airline pilots. That is Washington's little-used Dulles International, where you step aboard a ferry-like bus at your level and are driven from terminal to plane, or vice versa, and the bus is raised or lowered so its floor matches the one on which you're to step.

Since I have complained about the stairs on railroad cars, you might expect me to say the same thing about the loading or unloading stairs on the planes. I don't have the same complaints, for several reasons. The loading stairs used by most planes are not a part of the plane itself but are wheeled over to each plane as needed, so they are built with fairly gentle steps, not too high. The steps to get onto a railway car are part of the car itself, so they are built to be short and steep so as to take up as little space in the car as possible. Except for one plane, mentioned later, I don't find the normal boarding steps too difficult. Another difference, and it's a major one, is that the attitude of the carriers and their personnel is completely different. American railroads are doing their best to discourage passenger traffic, which is, generally, not profitable, and while individual conductors, porters, and trainmen may be nice and helpful, the over-all attitude is not too far from the "public be damned" statement attributed to an early railroader. The airlines are still trying to sell their service, to get passengers, and the employees are almost always courteous and helpful.

I rarely walk down an unloading stairway without someone from the airline walking backward in front of me, asking if he can help. That may just be care and courtesy, or it may be that employees have orders to do this so that no one will fall and sue the airline. As the planes get larger and larger, the entrances are often farther and farther from the ground when loading or unloading. On the other hand, the old DC-3, the last major commercial plane built before the universal adaptation of the tricycle landing gear, had a single wheel or skid at the rear, so when it was at rest on the ground there was a sharp slope inside the plane. The cabin floor was only a few steps off the ground, but it wasn't level once you got in until the plane took off. DC-3s are not a major problem for passengers today; the plane was phased out years ago, though some are still in use all over the world, mainly on local and feeder lines.

Generally, plane travel is made simple for the handicapped because the airlines go out of their way to make it easy. I have done a lot of flying on commercial airlines, domestic and foreign, and can make a personal generalization: the larger the airport, the bigger the airline, the better you'll be treated if you're handicapped. When the plane lands, I'm generally the last person out, as I don't want to hold up more agile and faster-moving passengers. On takeoff, I'm generally the first person on, as someone at the outgoing desk will notify me a few minutes before the gates are to be opened, so I can get on early and don't have to be in a crowd. I never ask for this; they just do it.

I like to sit far forward because it's usually smoother toward the front, and by a window, as I like to look out. But not in a seat by an emergency door, as my crutches may be taken from me so they won't block the exit. I like to keep them with me, as I can't move without them, but it's reasonable to require that they don't block an emergency exit. I've been on a few mildly hairy flights, all of which were concluded safely. Only once did my crutches cause any trouble, and then only to me. Years ago, on an Air France flight in Europe, a stewardess—not even a very pretty one—insisted that she had to take my crutches and would put them away and give them back to me when we landed. I thought I saw where she put them. But when we landed, she had disappeared and no one knew where they were or what I was talking about. I couldn't think of the French word for crutches *(béquilles)* and I could picture myself being stranded in that cabin. Eventually, someone found them for me. I make it a point, as a rule, to keep them within arm's reach. *My* arm.

Usually on domestic flights, when you emplane, you'll be asked whether you need help and would like a wheelchair when landing. Once or twice, I have used one. One time, I drove to the airport in a rented car with plenty of time to turn in the car and catch my flight, only to discover the car-rental place was empty. After waiting too long for someone to show up, I went to my airline office and explained my problem. As the car had been charged to my credit card, the airline girl took the keys and said she'd see it was taken care of, but as it was getting late I'd better go to the plane by wheelchair. So she called a porter and a wheelchair and had me pushed to the plane, whose entrance gate, as she knew, was a long way off.

I can also remember once getting into London's huge Heathrow Airport on a BOAC plane, planning to go elsewhere on a different airline an hour later. The other airline was about half a mile away. My baggage was transferred automatically, but I wasn't, so I stepped outside, called a taxi, and was driven to the other airline. At most big airports, you can catch an interior bus for such transfers, but at that time you couldn't in London. Even so, it would have been a question as to whether it would have been worth getting onto a bus. That would have depended on the type of step and entrance. Some of the interior airport buses are very easy to enter, with wide, low steps. At another European airport, the plane I was to take was pointed out to me, so far away it was but a small spot on the landscape. The airline decided the easiest way for me to get there was to put me in a wheelchair and push me to their own little ambulance with a lift gate, which lifted me, wheelchair and all, to the level of the interior of the plane so I could step right off and go to my seat.

The big commercial planes are pretty standardized by now, despite the advertising. Though there are some interior variations, depending on each airline's specifications, one 707 or DC-8 is very much like the next. Most travelers have their favorites for personal reasons. There is one short-range plane, however, that I don't like, the French Caravelle. It's a pleasant enough plane when flying, but the entrance and exit stairs—perfectly safe, I'm sure—are rickety and wobbly with a handrail that gives you no feeling of stability. A passenger who just runs up the stairs probably wouldn't notice it. The new wide-bodied jets, the 747s, DC-10s, and L-1011s, are higher off the ground than the old models, which makes them a little more work to enter or leave if you're not at an airport that uses jetways. They have more interior room once you're inside, which is sometimes a convenience, particularly for people traveling with small children. Their emergency or "crash" exits, however, are cloth sliding chutes, which might give me pause if I had to use one. I've never needed one and the chances are I never will. I hope not, for other reasons.

I've always found all the airlines extremely helpful and courteous, but only one seems to make a specific effort to go after the business of those who don't get around well, Pan American World Airways. Pan Am runs a series of tours for the physically disabled. In the past, these have included all-expense trips to the British Isles, Central Europe, the Middle East, Hawaii, and the Orient. Everything is worked out for the people who need canes, crutches, or wheelchairs to get about, including special buses for tripping or sightseeing, with a portable elevator to raise and lower passengers or wheelchairs. This is a comparatively new concept for Pan Am, which started these special tours in 1972 and found that, with very little publicity, they were selling out. They can be booked through Pan Am or most travel agents, generally at no extra cost.

Another service for handicapped travelers is offered by the car-rental firms. The two largest, Hertz and Avis, have equipment available for use by people who don't have the use of their legs or who need other special equipment. Hertz has hand-controlled cars for handicapped drivers in a dozen major cities, and will furnish them in other cities if given two days' advance notice. Avis asked for ten days' to two weeks' notice if the place where such a car is needed doesn't have these special cars available, which the local offices are supposed to be able to tell you. Neither firm charges extra for this special equipment.

After World War II, when automatic transmissions became generally available and there were many single and double amputees coming from the battlefields and hospitals, the federal government started providing certain disabled veterans with cars with automatic transmissions or hand controls if necessary. The city of New York, where parking is difficult at best and impossible at worst, met this problem by issuing SVI (Special Vehicle Identification) cards to drivers who qualified. I have had one for years, and would find it very difficult to live and work and travel in New York City the way I do if I didn't have my SVI shield.

They are issued by the Traffic Department, after a rather rigorous examination, including a report from your own doctor and an examination by a Police Department physician, as well as an investigation of your need for such a parking permit. The card has your name, license-plate number, and description on it, and after you have signed your name at the proper place, the card has to be encased in plastic so it cannot be altered. Usually, the card is placed on the sun visor, so it can be put out of sight when not needed and put down where it'll show when you are parking. This becomes so much a matter of habit that I found I was putting my visor down automatically when stopping in my garage. The SVI card enables the holder to park without fear of getting a valid ticket or being towed away in a no-parking zone, and lets him park without having to put coins in a parking meter. With the SVI shield comes a rear-bumper sticker to be attached near the license plate saying that a parking permit is in front, so a traffic policeman can see it before he writes out the license number to give you a ticket.

Despite this, I have received a good many parking tickets, usually given by a policeman who is giving them to a row of illegally parked cars in a street and has started to write the ticket before he sees the permit. As parking tickets in New York are numbered, once he has started to write it up he has to finish it, as it cannot be torn up. Today, there is a space on the summons for your SVI number so you can fill out the ticket and mail it in with your request to have it dismissed. Some time later, it will be mailed back to you, marked "Violation Dismissed, Valid Defense."

One of the troubles with having an SVI card is that your car may be stolen and sit unnoticed for ages because of it. My car was taken once, and about two weeks later the police called me to say they'd found it, many miles away. They picked me up in a prowl car and drove me to a remote area in the Bronx. Probably my car had been taken by some kid who used it one night and left it there. It was unhurt, just very dirty and dusty outside, as any car in New York would be, not moving for two weeks. It was on a street where without the SVI card it would have been ticketed in time, or possibly removed by the Sanitation Department. Or vandalized. I might add that I don't know whether it can be credited to the SVI card or not, but I have never lost even a hubcap in the city.

Most people don't know what the SVI card entitles the driver to do, or what it means. I had a neighbor who used to complain about my car being parked in front of his house. He used to complain by calling the Police Department. He didn't know that eventually the complaint would get to the SVI division and a friend there would call me and tell me old So-and-so was complaining again because the street was posted, no parking between eight A.M. and seven P.M. I didn't mind him complaining, it wasn't important to me. But I did mind his giving me the big, friendly hello right after he'd called and tried to get me in trouble. He lived in Manhattan, but had a country place in a different state and kept out-of-state license plates on his car, probably using his country place as his official residence so he didn't have to pay the high New York City insurance rates. One day when he had telephoned in a complaint and then given me a warm greeting, I told him to stop his complaints or I would report the out-of-state license on his Rolls. I never got another complaint. But I didn't like him any better either.

At one time I drove a rather large convertible. After a while, I stopped locking the car every time I got out. I didn't leave anything in it that could be stolen, putting everything in the trunk or the locked glove compartment. I stopped locking the car because sneak thieves would see the convertible and try to get into it by cutting the top, and new tops were expensive. Every now and then, the police would warn me about leaving my car unlocked, because someone might steal that SVI card. It wouldn't be useful to anyone else for any length of time, but people who didn't have them were envious and wouldn't know that just the possession of one wouldn't help much and would eventually get the illegitimate owner in trouble if he tried to use it.

I'm devoting a lot of space to this because that SVI card has been important to me. I have tried to explain that transportation, an independent form of transportation, is extremely important to the handicapped. The card has enabled me to use my car for my work and my pleasure in a way that would have been impossible without it. As is true with almost everything, of course, a part of its use depends on your own attitude. I've had nothing but the nicest, friendliest cooperation from the police. But a photographer I used to deal with, who walked with a good deal of difficulty, said he was always having fights with the police about his, every time he stopped. I didn't tell him that he had a real chip on his shoulder and was always having fights with everyone. As a matter of fact, I used him not because he was handicapped, but because, despite his personality, he was an excellent photographer.

I developed my own method for using the card. At any place where I parked regularly, I would find the policeman on the beat, explain that I was going to be there often, and ask where was it most convenient for him to have me leave my car. He always became my friend. At one publisher's, in a busy manufacturing area full of trucks parked on the streets for short periods while working, making pickups and deliveries, the traffic cop on the block was a mounted policeman and thus high enough to have a good picture of the parking situation. He would watch for me to arrive in the morning and, if there was no vacant place near my building, would tell me where I could find one, or even talk a truck driver into moving up a few feet to let me in. That was one reason why I didn't take the photographer seriously.

The same thing held true when I was covering first or second nights at the theater, in a normally jammed, no-parking area. I would find the mounted policeman on the street and ask where I should park. Invariably, he would ask what show I was going to see, and select a spot, and that would be that. I cannot recall a time when I have approached a policeman in New York and asked about parking that I wasn't treated with the utmost consideration. I would like to see all cities do something similar for their handicapped drivers. It can't be impossible; they have a model for it: New York, with little parking space and almost two million cars registered, has issued less than three thousand permits, and made life that much more pleasant for some of its citizens, without making it appreciably more difficult for the rest.

To the best of my knowledge, there has never been any corruption connected with these parking permits. New York

has more and worse problems than any other metropolis in
the country, due to the large number of people coming daily
into a limited area. Despite this, no other major city in the
country has done as much for its handicapped drivers. A list
of the activities of other big cities in the country is discouraging.

A few states issue special license plates to the physically
handicapped, but in general the parking privileges for the
users of these cars are limited by local law. Many cities that
allow parking privileges to the handicapped only permit
them to park for longer than the legally allowed time at
parking meters. Possibly the report from Washington, D.C.,
is the best brief explanation of how some communities feel
about the situation. The report said: no legislation, no provisions in any circumstances for special parking within the
street system, *no problems.* That's what the report says, no
problems. For whom?

Atlanta, Georgia, a growing, progressive city, has reported:
no legislation, no provisions for parking of handicapped per-
sons, special-permit privilege bill was introduced and de-
feated some years ago. Newark, New Jersey (whose handicapped can get New York SVI cards if they work in New York
City): no legislation, no provisions for on-street parking for
the handicapped, *no problems.* Houston, Texas: no city legislation, no state legislation, four authorized spaces set aside for
the handicapped at the fringe of the central business district.
Baltimore has set aside a total of six limited-parking zones for
the handicapped. Not six areas, but a space for a total of six
cars! Chicago has issued twenty-seven permits to handicapped vehicle operators, and parking for them is permitted
in designated areas as determined by the police.

The best thing that can happen to a physically handicapped person is for him to have a feeling of independence

and the confidence that comes from being able to get about, to go to work by himself, on his own. The big cities of the United States do very little for their handicapped in this respect, no matter what they may do in other fields.

CHAPTER NINE

The
Male-Female
Relationship

This may be the most important factor in the happiness of a handicapped person. In the life of anyone . . . relationships with those of the opposite gender.

It is of particular importance for the person with a physical handicap. He is apt to think his physical disability will hold him back in establishing or solidifying relationships with others—and if he doesn't think that, others will. As is the case with almost everything, the way this works out depends mainly on the person and his attitude.

For some reason I cannot understand, this has never been a problem for me. I'm not tall, dark, or handsome. I don't dance. Girls have never taken one look at me and started panting for my attention. It may be based on nothing but my conceit, but, despite surface handicaps, it has never occurred to me that any girl I wanted to get to know or take out wouldn't be glad to know me or go out with me. I know lots of men who can offer more in the way of youth, beauty, money, or laughter, but I've rarely been at a loss for women friends. I don't know why, but I've been on very friendly terms with many beautiful and talented women. In my opinion, to be attractive they had to be interesting to look at and be with, smart and original.

This all started quite early in my dating life, when I was barely in my teens. At that time, partying and dating were much more formal than today. Young men and young ladies went to parties, where dancing was a ritual. At some, girls had programs or cards and would be asked for certain dances, so the more popular girls had their cards filled up early. The dread of the less than very popular girl was being a wallflower, sitting alone or with other girls while the successful ones danced. The whole system was based on male supremacy in a form that seems laughable now, though it wasn't funny then, for some. I can't remember the first dance I went to or what happened, but I do remember that I developed a system very young: go after the prettiest and most popular girl at the party.

If this sounds childish, sophomoric, or shallow, it probably is, but it was also, in a sense, figured—based on observation. The girls who weren't the prettiest and most popular might not want to accept a nondancing date for a dance. If they were not out on the dance floor but sitting and talking to someone, people might think it was because no one had asked them to dance. Whereas the prettiest and most popular girl usually knew she was pretty and popular and knew that others knew it, too, so she had no hesitancy about accepting me as a partner. The seal of approval from the reigning belle automatically dispelled the doubts of the not-quite-reigning belles, too. I don't know just when I worked out that technique, but it was very early in my social life, and it worked. Once I discovered that, I didn't worry about parties and dances and the like, and when you don't worry about them, they're apt to go very much the way you'd like them to. One oddity is that I have always liked to watch dancing —ballet, ballroom, tap, any kind. When I was quite young and spending much time at the old Copley Plaza Hotel in Boston, it held regular tea dances and I used to go downstairs in the late afternoon and watch. It was this way, sitting in a wheelchair, that I got to know the fabulous Mrs. Jack Gardner of the house and art collection before she died. She liked to watch the dancers too.

An old friend, a newspaperman, recently said to me that I understood women, which was nonsense. Another person, a moderately aggressive young Women's Libber, at about the same time said I didn't have to learn any of this women's-equality stuff, and I realized what they both meant. I've always liked women, which may have been obvious by now in my references to my mother, sister, and grandmother, and I grew up in a family that respected them. I never thought women were to be considered as strange, different creatures. I was brought up to be polite to everyone, to speak gently, to hold doors and chairs for females and light their cigarettes, but otherwise treat them as people deserving respect or not, according to their individual qualities. I suppose this attitude showed and was appreciated. Conversely, some men I know whose behavior is most gallant and conspicuously polite secretly look down on women, and I think women see through it. At any rate, I've always gotten along well with women, and I'm glad, as it has made my life more pleasant.

While I'm against generalizations about people according to sex, color, religion, or ethnic background—I've never made a derogatory remark about a woman driver as such—

I have come to the conclusion that women, en masse, are less apt to behave considerately toward a handicapped male than are men. Singly and privately, women are, if anything, more considerate, but in a crowd it is different. The reason for this, in my opinion, has nothing to do with women as women, but is due to our culture. When I am bumped or jostled in a crowd, it is more apt to be by a woman than a man. I think this happens because women grow up expecting the man to give way to them, so they're not as careful about where and how they walk or move. Because many women expect men to perform small courtesies for them, they don't always react the way men do to certain situations, and that almost caused me mild trouble once.

There was a certain building in the Times Square area I used to go into and out of very often. It was a hectic sort of place in a hectic neighborhood, and it had heavy doors that opened with, or despite, strong springs. Many of the busy men going in or out, and seeing me coming, would hold the difficult door open for me. One day, as I was about to leave the building, a woman in front of me held the door for me, and I realized this had never happened there before. I thanked her, and as I had a car parked right outside the door —legally for me—I asked if I could offer her a lift. She looked at me as though I had suggested something very different and as though what she'd like to do was slap my face, said a short, "No," and hurried off. I could see her telling the story later: "I saw this poor guy and tried to help him by holding the door for him and he tried to pick me up!" I didn't—I was trying to thank her for a small courtesy, but she'd never believe that.

I've always felt that if you have to have a handicap, it's better to be a man than a woman. Generally, in our society, men have it better than women to start with. A physical handicap can be an economic disadvantage for a man, as it is usually figured that it is man's lot in the family to be the provider, but socially or sexually it is less of a disadvantage for a man than a woman to have a handicap like mine. A woman's legs are a part of her physical attraction, much more than a man's. As a matter of fact, I believe that the physical aspect of a woman is more important than that of a man, sexually speaking. But then, I'm not a woman and so I can't really tell. Until fairly recently, a woman with something wrong with her lower limbs couldn't very well hide it. Now women can and do wear pants, so they can hide braces or differences in size or shapeliness as men have been doing for years.

I think, too, that most men would be more apt to wonder about the physical or sexual capabilities of a handicapped woman than women would be to question a handicapped man. As a matter of fact, a handicapped man can use his handicap as a weapon against a reluctant woman. "You won't go out with me [or sleep with me] because I'm crippled." This is not an appeal I would ever use or think of. I picked it up listening to some men talking in a hospital and was amazed when I heard it. But, like much of such talk, it may have been a fantasy being verbalized.

The fear of a handicapped person that he will be sexually unattractive or incapable is something that sticks with the healthy as a possible nightmare. I realized this during and after World War II. I was toiling for the government, working six or seven days a week, ten or fifteen hours a day, when I received a phoned request from the Navy medical office in Washington asking me to go out to the naval hospital at St. Alban's on Long Island and see a certain doctor there. I did, and found it an interesting and worthwhile experience. The hospital was being used as a short-term assembly and distribution point for the severely wounded. These men would be flown in from Europe as soon as they could be moved, and then sent to the proper hospitals in the States, depending on the nature of their wounds, the type of treatment they needed, and the location of their homes and relatives.

I was supposed to go around the wards and talk to selected amputees and wounded. As a newspaperman, I was ostensibly interviewing them for articles to be sent to their local newspapers. That was my cover, and I used it. Actually, I was to answer their questions. I never found out who had suggested me for the job, nor was I curious, because I realized I could be useful in a way I should have thought of but hadn't. I was in my early thirties, which made me about ten years older than most of the men I interviewed. They were, in general, from small towns or farms in the Midwest or South, and not too well educated. They had one question they wanted to ask me. Not whether they would ever be able to walk or use their hands again, but how would they make out with the girls? This wasn't a question they could ask the nurses or doctors and get answers they believed.

They were full of doubts, the kinds and amounts depending on their physical and emotional status and maturity. A few were married; many had girls who were or were not "waiting" for them. The married, engaged, or spoken for all had the same worry: the girl in question, if she would have anything to do with them at all, would only be doing it out of pity. The ones who didn't have a girl—and these, of course, were usually the youngest—had different problems. Would they have a girl, ever? And why should they—what could they offer her?

Every time I went out there, I had a hard time getting away. Because I could only tell them that I had never had any trouble that way, that I had a wife and two lovely children.

I didn't say that the children were adopted because my wife had had a hysterectomy when she was twenty-two, because that had nothing to do with the case. After my first visit, I carried a small photo of my wife because she was a beautiful girl, and that seemed to please them. I also carried with me snapshots of the kids, because they were cute and pretty, but most little girls are cute and pretty. All I can say is that I felt my visits acted as a morale-booster, and if I was able to make one worried kid feel better about his problems, the time I spent was worthwhile. Though the hospital had a rapidly shifting population, my reputation seemed to go ahead of me. The staff would tell me whom I should see first, and various of the wounded were calling for me. I realized I was a small ray of light in a very dark and important time for them.

Not all of my visits were successful. I would run into a certain number of disbelievers, generally among the older men, often men who had prided themselves on their athletic ability and thought that was all that had made them sexually interesting. If I'm going to make any other generalization, it would be that the smarter they were, the easier it was to convince them that sexually their lives weren't going to be as changed as they had thought. Despite the occasional skeptic, I think my visits made the lives of those I saw a little more hopeful or less grim, and tended to make things easier later for their doctors, families, communities, and girls.

I've known a lot of men with physical handicaps, some of whom were successful in their relations with women, and some were not. I can say the same thing about men I've known without physical handicaps. To the best of my knowledge, I have never run into a handicapped male homosexual. That doesn't mean there aren't any—I just have never knowingly met any. The only handicapped homosexual I ever knew well was a woman. In her case, she said, it had begun early and was probably caused by fear. She was not a very attractive person, physically or mentally, and felt that she could never attract a nice man. Once I asked her why, if that was the case, she thought she could attract a nice woman. Her answer was so revealing and derogatory that it cut short the conversation: if she were a nice woman, she wouldn't be a Lesbian.

We were friendly for some months, until she moved to another part of the country for a new job. She told me once that I was the only man with whom she felt she could talk freely. When I asked her why, she said she felt that I was sympathetic and not sitting in judgment on her. In a way, that was true. I was sympathetic in that I felt sorry for her not because she was incapacitated but because she was unhappy. And I don't judge most people. I get along with people as a rule, and they tell me things. Partly because I listen and want to know. Whatever the reason, a large number of people have told me a good deal about themselves, and still do.

I've known a good many women with physical handicaps, and the same thing can be said about them as about the men: some of them have been able to lead remarkably full and productive lives, some have not. The ones who have been what I would call successful have been those who have made a specific effort to be attractive, to look their best. But that is a subjective judgment—it may be that is the type I like so I think they are successful.

I know a woman, attractive, bright, traveled, and popular. She has everything except two hands: one is missing. It is not something you notice. I remember being at her house once for a small party. She was expecting a new boy friend, and left the room and changed her clothes. She came back in very quickly, wearing a different outfit and, I noticed, a different glove. I commented on it and she took me to her bedroom, opened a bureau drawer, and said, "Look." It was jammed with gloves of different types and colors. It would have stocked the glove department of a store, except I am afraid they were all one size.

"I don't like to be any more noticeable than I have to," she said, "so I always wear gloves, or a glove, to match my dress."

All I can say is that this was a person with a mild physical problem that a stranger might notice but would forget almost at once because she seemed to pay so little attention to it. It was a mild physical problem because she made it totally unimportant. I noticed, for instance, that when eating out she always ordered food she could cut with a fork. A small thing, but one of the ways she didn't call attention to her missing hand. Otherwise, she seemed to ignore what might have been a problem.

Some people have problems they can't ignore, so they use them. I once knew a woman, thin and gifted, at least two inches over six feet in height. Knowing she would be taller and thinner than most, no matter how she tried to camouflage it, she decided to play it up, so she started wearing tight, vertically striped clothes and hats like shakos. It worked for her. Instead of being an extremely tall, slightly gawky-looking woman, she was a striking woman.

I know another woman who lost a leg long after she'd been married and raised a couple of children. She's a lovely and charming person. The thing you remember about her is that she seems so nice and so interested and so much at ease, not that she has one leg and goes around with crutches. She has said that her crutch pads automatically match her clothes; she would no more think of using crutch pads that didn't match what she was wearing than she'd think of going shopping without wearing anything.

Like many people who were incapacitated long after their habits had been formed, she had to make an adjustment she would have thought impossible earlier. For a few years, she thought her life was over; she would continue living, of course, but not with any pleasure in her life. It's an understandable reaction but one she looks back on now with a certain amount of astonishment and shame. At that time, if she hadn't already had children, she wouldn't have had any; she didn't think she would be able to take care of them. She didn't think she'd be able to take care of herself, much less a husband and a household.

She seems to be a happy, well-adjusted person, busy with all kinds of activities involving her family and community interests. You think of her only as a busy, interesting, involved woman. Judging from externals, she leads a more than normally satisfying life. I don't know anything about her sex life, but she seems to have a good relationship with her husband. One thing we rarely know about others is the quality of their sex lives because that is not a thing most people talk about very often or truthfully, unless for some reason or other it has a spectacular aspect.

While it is a most important aspect of everyone's life, it may be even more important for the handicapped because he or she may have abnormal worries about being able to lead a normal or satisfactory sex life, and because he or she is conscious that others may be wondering about it. Whether or not they will lead sexually satisfactory lives depends upon many factors not related to their handicaps. As any divorce lawyer, marriage counselor, or psychiatrist can tell you, large numbers of seemingly normal men and women have sexual problems and hangups. Whether or not a handicapped person has them depends largely on his attitude toward life, toward his handicap, and particularly toward himself.

Most people with unhappy sex lives don't like themselves

very much; they underrate themselves in comparison with others. This goes for the handicapped as well. A handicapped man or woman has a seemingly convincing reason for feeling he or she doesn't have the same things to offer one of the opposite sex that the next person has. This can have any number of effects: it can make him withdrawn and unsure, it can make him come on too strong, it can make him unselective. A large number of men and women fear they are not specially favored physically or socially and try to bolster sagging egos by making many conquests. That is the way they look upon their adventures, and the choice of the word "conquest" shows a bit of what is wrong with their sex lives.

Any kind of proper involvement with anyone of the other sex is a matter of give and take, of giving of yourself and accepting the giving of the other. It sounds simple, and is when it works, and it is pitiful and amazing how many people are unable to do it because they think they have to keep a firm grip on their precious selves. This causes enough trouble for people without a physical handicap. It can cause even more for the handicapped, because a person with this type of handicap is not as apt to meet as many people, of the opposite sex or not, as someone physically more active. That is a simple matter of physical activity and numbers. The more you get around, the more people you're apt to know; the more people you know, the more apt you are to meet someone you like or with whom you have a good deal in common.

There is usually no reason for physically handicapped people not to have a satisfactory love life, or romantic attachments, or whatever you want to call them on whatever level your taste dictates. From a standpoint of sex, the center of sexual activity, male or female, is not in the genitals; it is in the mind.

It has been my theory for many years that because I pay very little attention to my own physical problem, other people tend to forget it, too. To the best of my knowledge, it has worked out that way. The connection of sex and a physical handicap led to an odd experience years ago when I was in college.

I normally had dinner at one particular table in a corner of the dining hall, with half a dozen classmates. It wasn't a formal arrangement, we ate together because we liked one another. Someone going down to dinner would stop and see if the others were planning to eat, and we'd always eat at the same table because one of our little group was getting his meals without cost by waiting on that table. No matter what our activity or schedule was, we always knew that if we arrived within certain hours we would find friends at that table.

One night, I was sitting in the corner, as usual, so my crutches could stand within reach, out of the way, at the juncture of two walls. We were joined this night by a comparative stranger, a student none of us knew except to nod to as a fellow student. He asked if he could join us, and did. Somehow the conversation turned to a character suddenly prominent in the news: a man with a noticeable limp, who might even have been nicknamed The Gimp, had disappeared with a famous beauty. The stranger made a number of stupid and tasteless remarks about this that were mildly embarrassing in the circumstances, not to me but possibly to him if and when he realized that the crutches in the corner belonged to someone at the table.

"You've got to watch these cripples, you know. They're sexy as hell. If the blood can't go to their legs in the regular way, it has to go someplace. . . ." (This, incidentally, is a fairly common notion. I knew a one-legged foreign correspondent who did pretty well by spreading that story.) At any rate, I decided the thing to do was sit at the table until the stranger finished eating and talking and left. But he said so many stupid and annoying things that it looked as though they could go on forever, so I nudged one of my friends and said, "Let's go." I reached for my crutches and got up, waving a casual "See you" to the stranger and walked away.

One of our friends who had come in late told me afterward that the stranger had turned purple and asked, "Why didn't you tell me, why didn't you stop me?" My friend said he'd answered, "Look, you were talking stupidly. I know Joe well, and know he'd only find this funny, and if you wanted to dig a hole for yourself with your mouth, you deserved to fall in for being so thoughtless. Suppose it had been someone who would have been hurt or upset."

I am reminded of a similar, nonhandicapped incident that took place at a formal dinner many years later. The strange lady at my left suddenly asked me, during one of those lulls in the conversation that let everyone hear what is being said across the table, "You're Mr. Marx? You're not by any chance related to that old battle-ax Blanche Marx, are you?" That happens to be my mother's name, and while she is a bright, intelligent, and charming woman, she has a dynamic and vivid personality and could rub someone the wrong way who held opposing views. There was a total silence in the dining room before I answered. I thought not of defending my mother, who doesn't need it, but that anyone stupid enough to make a remark like that to a total stranger deserved what she got, so I said, "Yes. She's my mother."

At one time, I lived for a few years in a small town (7,000) in the southern Midwest, becoming very friendly there with a blind lawyer, a man who had lost his sight when he was about twelve. Despite that, he had gone to Harvard College and the Harvard Law School. Living in a small town and prevented from traveling freely alone, he had been married at different times to three lovely women when I lost track of him. I mention this because you might think a blind man living in a small town would have trouble finding one wife, much less three women from widely separate parts of the country. The reason was simple: he was an unusual and interesting man, and he had something to offer. Not his eyes, but a mind, and sensitivity, and courtesy, and consideration.

I had liked him from the time I had met him, when we had attended a concert in a neighboring city. It happened that we were the only males in our little group at the concert, and during intermission when my new friend wanted to go to the men's room he asked me to guide him. We were walking across the crowded hall, with his hand on my shoulder for guidance, when he suddenly chuckled and said, "This is sort of the classic situation, isn't it?" That was the beginning of a good friendship.

The only thing I could do to simplify his life was make it a point that each time he came to our house, every bit of furniture was exactly where it had been the last time he had visited. He used to worry me at times when I visited him because his hobby was woodworking and he used power tools. You'd go to his house and call out for him and hear his machinery going. It was an unreasonable surprise to find him in his basement workroom with various pieces of machinery running and no lights. He made some very pretty things, too. We were good friends for some years. I was quite impressed by him because he had made so much of a life for himself despite what might have been considered a most severe handicap.

The handicapped, like others, will run into a certain number of people who are sick or disturbed. I used to know a rather bright, attractive young man who had a string of girl friends, none of whom lasted very long with him. It wasn't until I met the third or fourth one that I realized there was a pattern—they all had some kind of physical problem, a missing or deformed part of their anatomy. He stayed in this pattern for some years and suddenly took up with, and married, a lovely, bright girl who had nothing at all wrong with her, mentally or physically. Since then, they've had a couple of children, and, as far as I know, he has gotten over his aberration.

I cannot stress enough the principle that a loving or sexual relationship does not have to be based on physical perfection. Not even a commercial sexual relationship. I was once quite friendly as an editor with a hard-working Midwestern prostitute. I never met her, but we corresponded regularly for years and she sent me some good material. She wrote me once about a one-legged girl she had worked with in a "house." The girl wouldn't work in a place where she had to climb upstairs to get to her room with her client—that wasted too much of her time and energy. But she used the fact that she had only one leg as a form of come-on. "Ever try it with a one-legged girl?" she asked. "Try it now. Change your luck," she would tell a potential customer. Reportedly, it worked well for her—some customers were repelled by the idea, but others were intrigued. That was a handicapped person trying to keep a physical handicap from interfering with her form of making a living by what must be called physical work.

There is no good reason for most handicapped people not to marry. Often they marry late, a fairly high percentage well after the usual marriage age. One reason is opposition or discouragement from prospective in-laws. Many a parent who would put up only token opposition to a child's marriage will take a much stronger stand if the new member of the family has a physical handicap. This is often based on real or imagined problems about money-making capacity or general usefulness.

A man whose daughter is getting married wants to feel that his child will be taken care of, protected as much as possible. If the prospective husband is going to have trouble making a living, that is one problem. If, in addition, he will be unable to do much of the heavy physical work that goes with some homemaking, that is an additional problem to be considered.

A man whose son is marrying a handicapped girl has another angle to the same problem. What kind of a house will she be able to run? How can she do the marketing, cleaning, cooking usually considered to be part of the wife's role? Will she be able to have children? If so, will she be able to take care of them? These are questions that plague the minds of parents, and also figure in the plans and considerations of those who are getting married.

Another reason for late marriage among the handicapped is economic. It usually takes longer for a handicapped person to get a job or find a vocation than for one without his particular problems . . . and when he does get one, it probably will not be as high-paying. These are physical and economic problems. Add to these the psychic problems. A young handicapped person often does not put a high enough value on his own worth to allow him to become emotionally involved in a serious manner with another. A girl may not be sure of her ability to have or raise children. But then, as they grow older, they realize that they can do many of the tasks they worried about and find ways around some of the others, and that many of the problems are not as serious as they had seemed earlier.

That goes for what might be called a mixed marriage, in which one of the partners has a handicap while the other is physically normal. But what about two handicapped people —should they marry? And does it happen often?

There is something to be said on each side of this question. First of all comes the simple universal problem of love. If they love each other enough, they will probably find a way to make it work. If they don't, it probably wouldn't work in any case. The physical handicap should not be the determining factor, once the couple knows what the problems are and faces them. I am taking it for granted that they are sexually compatible. Individually each will have become accustomed to having been a center of attention just because of being different. Now as a couple they will get much more attention, as well as becoming objects of curiosity. They must be pretty sure their feelings for each other are strong enough to stand up under it.

They will have to consider the physical problems of their joint handicaps. Will either of them be able to lift and carry? Can they work it out together? What about the usual tasks that have to do with living—can they work out a pattern so that they can divide these tasks according to what each can do?

There are no specific answers to many of these questions, because, as in any question about any marriage, it all depends . . . In the case of two handicapped people marrying, it depends on the nature of the handicaps and the adjustments that have been made and will or can be made. As is true of many complications, they can be eased if there is plenty of money. Money to buy or rent the kind of living space that their *joint and individual* handicaps can function in. Money to provide the type of help they may need in order to function.

These are just some of the problems that have to be faced rationally. Exact answers are not easy because there are so many ifs. But, in general, if two handicapped people can honestly face up to the problems and still want to take their chances and get married, the world should say: More power to them.

It happens often enough. Not necessarily because handicapped people, male and female, are attracted to each other by some psychic or mystic bond, but because people tend to meet and marry their counterparts, millionaires or paupers, Frenchmen or Scots, Hindus or Republicans. As the rich tend to go around with the rich, and thus meet more of the opposite sex who are rich and marry them, so the handicapped are often thrown together, in hospitals, clinics, schools, jobs. Once they work out the basic special problems that confront them, they usually make a pretty good job of marriage.

After all, they should. They usually marry later, and with their eyes wide open, not full of moon dust. On the average, if their marriages worked out as badly as the usual marriage, it would be pretty disappointing.

CHAPTER TEN

Hospitals, Doctors, and Nurses

Hospitals, usually imposing, clean-looking buildings, are a major and noticeable part of our cities. They should be. Most citizens use them many times in a lifetime. A few simple statistics show how important they are in the life of the average man, woman, and child. In 1971 (the last year for which I have figures, and these figures don't change much from year to year), there were 7097 hospitals in the United States, of which 407 were federal, leaving 6690 to be utilized by and paid for by others. The federal hospitals admitted 1,788,000 patients, the nonfederal ones took in 30,875,000 ailing people, making a total of 32,663,000.

The only purpose in giving these statistics is to show that one out of every six or seven people in the United States was admitted to a hospital as an in-patient during the year. Statistics, while interesting, rarely tell the whole story, except to insurance companies. All they can divulge are over-all figures, not what happens to an individual. Most handicapped people have spent considerable time in hospitals, with results varying from miraculous to terrible. These results depend on the hospital, the disease, the doctor, the patient, the nurses, and luck, not necessarily in that order. I started young and have spent more time than most in hospitals and dealing with doctors and nurses. They all differ from one another, as you might expect, the way other people and things do.

And, as other people and things do, they sometimes fail to live up to their public image. The great white (or gray) house of mercy may in fact be an overly expensive, inefficiently run haven for educated, bureaucratic bunglers. The kindly, knowledgeable physician may be a stupid, neurotic man or woman who will do you more harm than good before overcharging you. The kindhearted, dedicated nurse may be a lazy harpy who doesn't give a damn about you or how you feel and devotes most of her waking time to thoughts about her own paycheck and ways to improve it. Mind you, not all who treat the ill are like this, but enough medical buildings and people match the above descriptions to make them a problem for the others, as well as for the patients.

If the above sounds as though I'm bitter, I'm not. I have been extraordinarily well treated by hospitals, doctors, and nurses. But then, I'm an experienced patient, which helps, and I'm white, English-speaking, not illiterate, and soft-spoken, which helps, too. I've been lucky in my relations with the medical profession. But I've been lucky with auto mechanics, too, which is not pure dumb luck. I did study engineering, and I know the principles on which automobiles run, and like making my own repairs. If this comparison insults either profession, it's not meant to, but it has some validity. There are fine people in each profession, but not all doctors or mechanics are fine. As a patient, I have gotten to know a good many doctors, both professionally and personally, and as an individual, I've come to know a good many more. I like some, admire some, and dislike some. They share the good and bad traits of all people, sometimes exaggerated.

There was a time when the men who followed a medical career were generally admired and looked up to. Despite doctors' opinions of themselves, that time has long since passed. And despite the popularity of medical shows on television and such mythical practitioners as Marcus Welby, the general feeling about doctors, their efficiency, knowledge, and over-all goodness, has slipped in the public's esteem just as the reputation of lawyers has. And for much the same reason: they began to believe their own press clippings, they saw themselves as selfless creatures serving the public at great personal inconvenience.

This picture is a true portrait of some doctors. It is also true of some attorneys. There is much to be said for the medical profession. The trouble is that it isn't as one-sided as doctors and the AMA would have you believe. It's not easy to become a doctor and be licensed to practice medicine in the United States. It takes a good deal of time, energy, money, work, and sometimes even brains. But, despite this, not all doctors are smart or well trained, any more than all members of any other profession. Some are just smart enough to learn how to give the right answers to get them grades good enough to get through med school. Then they have to go through more years of training, of internship and residency in a hospital and other forms of what might be termed apprenticeship. By the time they are able to be working on their own and in their chosen field, they have usually lost the first blush of youth along with their youthful idealism and enthusiasm.

I've known some doctors who were extraordinarily able men, dedicated and capable in their work and almost saintly in their character. And some who were fine men medically and sadly lacking as human beings. I've known others who were excellent mechanics, who regarded the human body as a mechanism that occasionally or habitually got out of order and could be treated like a balky piece of plumbing or a stalled automobile engine, and with just about as much human feeling. These doctors have their uses, too, depending on why they're needed. Some of the coldest doctors make excellent surgeons, for instance. As medical knowledge and techniques havé advanced in quantum jumps, doctors have had to go in more and more for specialization and have tended to live up to that old definition of a specialist: one who knows more and more about less and less.

The old-fashioned horse-and-buggy doctor, the general practitioner, the old Family Doctor who made calls in any weather and at all hours, seems to have disappeared like the passenger pigeon. He might not have fitted at all into a modern America. But he had one great advantage: he knew his patients and usually knew their families, too. This is something that generally is missing in the modern computerized, specialized practice. Many of today's doctors seem to have forgotten that a patient doesn't live in a vacuum but is part of a family, and what is best for the patient has to be considered in the context of what will be best for the family as a whole, not just one individual.

A successful doctor has to walk a fine line between getting so involved with his patients that he cannot function efficiently and becoming so impersonal that his efficiency has less than its full effect. A certain loss of sensitivity is a development that often takes place with age and experience, because the young doctor was too thoughtful and considerate and spent too much of himself because of his empathy with his patients. This could reach a point where it interfered with his work, with his ability to sleep or relax, where it became detrimental to his judgment and mechanical ability and dexterity. This, in turn, often resulted in a deliberate pulling back, a stifling of human feelings, which may make for a more efficient doctor but something less of a human being.

Harry Truman used to have a sign on his desk in the White House reading: THE BUCK STOPS HERE. A politician can often duck the responsibility for certain difficult decisions, but there are some things a President has to decide in a clear-cut fashion. Despite the growth of group medicine, consultations, and the like, doctors early learn that they have to make decisions; that in many cases the decisions cannot be based on the definite results of tests but have to be based on that combination of experience and intelligence we often call intuition; and that the decision will determine whether someone will live or die. Having to decide repeatedly and successfully gives many doctors a sort of "God complex." They have to believe they're right or they'd lose their reason. They are often surrounded by admiring assistants, younger doctors, trainees, and the like who add their adulation to the ambience of omnipotence in which the doctor moves.

Among other factors contributing to this is the fact that wealth is respected, and in most cities and towns the successful doctors are among the community's leaders financially and otherwise. In spite of all their cries about the work they do for charity, and many of them do a good deal of it, if you look around an average city or town in almost any part of the country, you'll find very few poor doctors, unless they're very young. And several wealthy doctors among the town's upper-income elite. This often adds to the doctor's feeling of superiority, which can be replaced by one of infallibility, a process at times abetted by the attitude of the American Medical Association. Attendance at a convention of the AMA would be instructive for most patients, just as reading a publication like *Medical Economics* would be useful.

The profession of medicine is generally respected among the wealthy as well as the underprivileged. It isn't only the daughter of the fabled Jewish mother who is considered to have made a good match if she marries a doctor. This holds true throughout the country and goes through the mores of almost all ethnic groups. A medical convention will consist of many learned papers and discussions on technical and esoteric subjects (except to the specialists in that field) and just as much gossiping about lucrative posts, good investments, and tax shelters as you'll find at a convention of bankers.

Medical Economics goes out free to every recognized doctor in the country, and carries more advertising than most periodicals. The magazine is a good, professional job and makes a good deal of money for its publishers. Its emphasis is just what the title says. While it often carries articles on new developments in medicine, like the more authoritative *Journal of the American Medical Association,* the bulk of the editorial content consists of articles giving doctors useful tips on how to improve their earnings or keep-home pay. Articles on how much to charge for certain services and how to figure them, on how to collect from slow patients without losing their patronage, on the latest tax wrinkles and how to take advantage of them. There is nothing wrong or even vaguely dishonest about this. But for those who believe in the propaganda of the AMA, the print order, profits, and advertising and editorial content of *Medical Economics* would come as an eye-opener.

Most people believe, and want to believe, that their doctor is the greatest, the best. That is useful for them as patients.

Unless a patient believes his doctor knows what he is doing, he isn't going to benefit much from following his doctor's advice. I've been lucky in knowing so many doctors on a personal basis; I could see them as individual people and usually have been treated by them as a person, not a case.

I've had to go to many doctors for many reasons, but mainly in this book I'm talking about two orthopedic surgeons in Boston who did so much work on me. The first was Dr. Robert Lovett, a tall, dignified, starchy man who was selected by my parents after a wide search. They operated on the theory that, after a major epidemic, one man will emerge preeminent in that field. Dr. Lovett was highly regarded after a polio epidemic in the Northeast. Of course, he had been highly regarded before it, but it was afterward that we heard of him. He was head of the orthopedic section of the Harvard Medical School and, as far as I was concerned, a delightful and wonderful man. As he grew older, his chief assistant, Dr. Frank Ober, took over more and more of his work and in due time succeeded to his post at Harvard. Both of them knew me and worked on me from the time I was a child until they died.

One of their better-known patients was Franklin D. Roosevelt, who hadn't had polio at the time I went to them. I remember that when I saw *Sunrise at Campobello*, a play and movie about how FDR came down with polio and later overcame it enough to run for President, I was intrigued by two things. The first was a line early in the play when Sara, FDR's mother, heard the news of her son's illness and immediately asked whether anyone had sent for Dr. Lovett.

The other minor point that caught my attention was watching Ralph Bellamy, playing Roosevelt, learn to walk again, using crutches. I watched in agony because he was making mistakes and they would cause him to fall. And they did, until he learned how to manipulate them properly. Dr. Lovett, as befitted his attainments and the number of people clamoring for his attention, was regarded not only as a minor deity but as something of a dictator. Except by me, for behind his stern, autocratic manner I saw a man with humor and kindness, and a man who loved and felt for children.

His office took up a medium-sized private house at 234 Marlboro Street in the Back Bay section of Boston, and had quite an elaborate routine so the great man could give his personal attention to as many people as possible. There was a large staff of doctors, nurses, physical therapists, secretaries, and the like. As a patient, you would be taken over by members of the staff to be weighed, measured, and have various muscles and reactions tested and compared with previous tests. Eventually, the great man would appear with his small entourage, and everyone would fall silent so the doctor in charge of the preliminaries could report findings. Dr. Lovett would listen, ask questions, talk to the patient, and decide what was to be done next.

One time, when Dr. Lovett appeared, I was deep in a discussion about stamps with a young doctor, and Dr. Lovett asked the assistant a question about my progress. I said, "Could you wait a minute? We were talking about something very important." The young doctor was embarrassed; the group was shocked and waited for the lightning to strike. But Dr. Lovett put his hand on my head and said, "Go right ahead, Joe, and finish your talk." So I did, as the young doctor hurriedly brought it to an end. I should have felt ashamed of holding up the busy man, but I wasn't—he understood, as I knew he would. I was maybe ten years old, and what we had been discussing was important to me; examinations by doctors were routine.

Being on good terms with Dr. Lovett came in handy later.

I had been operated on at Boston's Children's Hospital, and was in there for some time. I was ambulatory after a fashion —I was able to move around in a chaise type of a wheelchair. After being there a few weeks, I was bored with the food. Institutional food of any kind is not apt to be interesting. At the time at that hospital, it had its own pattern of dullness, because the menu was the same for each specific day of the week. Monday's dinner was the same as last Monday's and next Monday's. This made it easier for the hospital to plan, purchase, and prepare meals. But when you're recuperating in a hospital, meals are important breaks in the day. Being by nature a quiet sort of activist, I visited all the other long-term patients on my floor and organized a hunger strike. We would stop eating until they made some menu changes.

We did, and somehow one of the newspapers heard about it and our hunger strike became a mini *cause-célèbre*. Dr. Lovett took it up with me, and I explained why I'd started it. He gave me the hospital's position, but said he'd check out the standardized menus and speak to the hospital about putting a little variety into them. He must have, because the menus started to change and we called off the strike.

What was done to me at that hospital then was a series of operations on my right leg, then the bad one, misshapen and almost useless. Dr. Lovett was transferring and transplanting muscles and rebuilding a foot and leg. After a time, he succeeded. It not only worked, but once I learned how to operate the transplanted muscles, I could move my leg and foot in all directions. In rebuilding my right foot, Dr. Lovett had even given it a nice, clear but delicate arch. He was very proud of that job, and once every so often when I was in Boston, he would borrow me for an evening for use as an exhibit to the students at Harvard Med. Instead of a chalk talk, I was a living lecture exhibit. It was so impersonal that I rather liked it.

After Dr. Lovett died, it came as no surprise to anyone that he was succeeded by Dr. Ober. Two more different men would be hard to imagine. Dr. Lovett was tall, thin, aloof, and austere, a picture of the perfect Bostonian of a classic type. Dr. Ober was a large man, ample of girth. While I could discern the twinkle in Dr. Lovett's eyes, and probably took advantage of my knowledge that it was there, everyone could see and hear Dr. Ober's deep chuckle. Dr. Ober, succeeding Dr. Lovett both at Harvard and as FDR's doctor, continued with Dr. Lovett's large practice. Dr. Ober had been born and raised on Mount Desert Island, off the coast of Maine. As an independent State of Maine man, he created something of a rumpus when he was put on the board of governors of the AMA.

He explained it to me once. "Because I tried to do something so that people who couldn't afford our services wouldn't have to be treated as charity patients, I was accused of trying to foster what they called socialized medicine. You see, Joe, in the old days, when a man had trouble, if his house or barn burned down, his neighbors would take some time off and pitch in and help, and together they'd build a new one. Today, we live in a different type of society, so we have to use a different method to obtain the same ends."

It was a typical Down East way of expressing things. I've never known whether his social philosophy would have evolved the way it did if he had been just a conventional, successful orthopedist or whether it had been affected by his long, close contact with Franklin Roosevelt. His more conservative co-workers may have thought the latter. Perhaps his heresy was that he was more interested in his work and his fellow man than in his own profit. He was never known as a man who sent small bills to people who could afford to pay large ones, but few, if any, of his less affluent patients considered him a money-grubber.

Among doctors in general, I have rarely met any group who seem kinder or more dedicated to the best ideals of their profession than those orthopedic and rehabilitation specialists who devote themselves mainly to pediatrics. There seems to be something about a crippled child that brings out the best in most people, and those medical men and women who devote themselves to working with children seem to form an especially fine group.

I've always gotten along well in hospitals. I don't like to be in them unless I'm desperately ill, but they're easy to get along in once you learn to fit yourself into their routine instead of trying to get them to bend to fit your preferences. The only time I ever had any trouble in a hospital was caused inadvertently by Dr. Ober being nice to me. He had operated on me in New York and, when his current patients were recuperating, went back to Boston, to return in a week or two. Trying to make things pleasant for me, he told the staff that he was leaving no instructions with them for treatment of me—"Joe knows as much about procedure as I do, and more about himself"—and went back to his home base. That sounded fine, but didn't work out well.

Most hospitals, and the nurses in charge, don't like to be told what to do by a patient. They're accustomed to being instructed by doctors—whom they can respect or not, depending on their opinion of the doctor—but not by patients. I don't think that Dr. Ober, trying to make things easy for me, realized the power that the nursing staff holds over patients. By the time he came back to New York, we had worked it out, but the nurses were unhappy until they realized that I wasn't arbitrary and had no intention of doing anything contrary to their customs and regulations, which I knew by that time. The well-being and comfort of a patient is in the hands of the hospital staff; his state of mind and physical comfort are affected by the way he is treated by nurses, aides, orderlies, and the like much more than by the doctors. Patients and staff members realize this; most doctors don't seem to, though many pay lip-service to the principle.

Hospitals are unavoidably inefficient. In most places, it costs more than $100 a day to stay in one. One of the reasons for the high cost is that the patient is paying for equipment and services that usually are not needed but, when they are, are needed desperately, often being able to make the difference between life and death. If you've ever seen a good hospital, or section of one, mobilize for an emergency, you've seen men and women at their best, working together efficiently and selflessly. Otherwise, hospitals seem to muddle along, doing their best. Few patients are there because they like being in a hospital. They are there because they're too sick to stay home, and there may be no place else where they can get any care, much less the kind of care they need.

Most hospitals are run on rigid routines that seem to have been set up for the convenience of the staff rather than the patients. There are many layers of bureaucrats managing hospitals, and how well each hospital runs depends more on the efficiency of the people than of the system. As a patient, you may have trouble sleeping or getting to sleep, but most patients are awakened from one to three hours earlier than their normal at-home waking time. There are a number of reasons for this, not unsound and mainly concerned with the people working there. The early waking hour lets the hard-working day shift come on duty after the night shift has done a good deal of the preparatory work, getting the patients awakened, freshened up a bit, fed, often bathed and equipped with fresh linen. By the time the outside doctor comes to pay his morning call, you and your room and cellmate or mates are in fair condition, your charts have been brought up to date, and interns and residents have done the necessary chores. So you're able, with luck, to answer the doctor and describe your symptoms, to withstand the rigors of the day and what he intends to do with you. The day may begin, chronologically, with the noisy crack-of-dawn awakening, but the real day doesn't begin until the doctor's visit.

Hospitals are usually difficult, physically, for the aged, infirm, or weak to get into. The imposing buildings often have a few steps to climb and then heavy swinging doors on strong springs to open, or even heavier revolving doors to get through. Unless one is sick enough to be carried or wheeled in via the ambulance entrance, just getting inside the building can be a wearing task. In almost any hospital, you can pick up at least one horror story about some recent dreadful mistake. This is not necessarily the fault of the hospitals; they are run by people and thus subject to human error. The trouble with hospitals as they are now is that we haven't found anything better to take their place.

They aren't supposed to be, but often are, rather complex contradictions. The operating rooms may have complicated machinery for sterilizing the air and everything else so that an opened-up patient may stay healthy and aseptic, but the working lower basements can be filthy, a condition that may or may not be dangerous to patients. Trays come from the kitchens with carefully color-coded cards so that patients on certain diets will get food that is right for them in their condition . . . and then are served to the wrong eaters. Most patients survive without realizing the error, because usually people are basically healthier than they are given credit for and one wrong meal isn't going to do too much damage.

It is not easy to see how many of the hospital costs can be reduced, since really efficient utilization of equipment is not possible because a hospital, by its nature, has to be equipped for emergencies. The nature of the emergency cannot be forecast with any accuracy. Certain items can be calculated because of location, climate, the nature of the predominant industries in the area, and similar factors. A hospital in a mining or heavy-industry town will not have to treat the same kind of injuries as one in an agricultural or light-industry area. But random incidents occur. A blood bank can tell from experience the amount of each different type of blood it will probably use in a specified period, and then will run into a week or a month when the requests for one specific type of blood are double the normal amounts.

Hospitals in a city or area will cooperate on equipment, borrowing from each other, sometimes by plane, unusual or rare types of medicine, serums, or vaccines, as well as machinery. Emergencies of this type are usually caused by an epidemic, accident, or natural disaster. In large metropolitan areas, certain hospitals may in time specialize in one type of medicine. I don't mean the ones whose names show that they are concentrating on problems connected with sight or hearing or births, but general hospitals that get a reputation for a certain type of medicine or surgery. Sometimes, this is planned to fill a need; more often, it comes about because a brilliant practitioner in one field happens to be there. This, in turn, attracts more doctors who specialize or would like to specialize in that field.

If people could be sorted out and classified and sent to the hospitals with the best equipment for their needs, much trouble and expense could be avoided. Only the Veterans Administration seems capable of doing this on a nationwide basis, and it does so in many instances. It has a certain number of specialized hospitals to which some of its patients can be sent for advanced care. But, for most people, the nearest local hospital, or the one their doctor uses, is the one to which they'll go. People don't fit neatly into categories, and neither do their ailments.

In order to become a psychoanalyst in many states, the would-be shrink first has to get his M.D., then take other courses and go through psychoanalysis. Hospitals might be better places for most patients if doctors had to go to them as patients. It wouldn't work, of course, as they still wouldn't be treated the way most patients are—they would automatically be favored and privileged. I don't wish any doctors any bad luck or illnesses, but it might do some good. Every now and then a doctor or a member of a doctor's family is treated the way other patients are, and all hell breaks loose. As I've said, I have always been treated nicely, and usually admire the hospitals, their results, and the people who work in them.

In many hospitals, a quiet, unseen war is being waged continually, like that between the bridge and the engine room on a ship. In a hospital, it is between the hospital administration and the medical staff. Sometimes this works for the patients' benefit, keeping both sides on their toes; sometimes it makes for unhappiness and bitterness. The most important part of a hospital does not consist of its medical staff or its buildings and equipment. It is an intangible thing: the spirit of its staff. If a patient is going to be in a hospital for any length of time, he realizes that his comfort depends less on the doctors, interns, residents, and registered nurses than it does on the student nurses, the nurses' aides, the paramedical help, the assistants and orderlies, and the domestics, the cleaning men and women. If they get along with each other, if they seem to like their work and their surroundings, the patient is going to feel and be well treated.

Nurses and nurses' aides are most important in the smooth running of any hospital. Nurses, like doctors and patients, come in all sizes and shapes, physically and temperamentally. I've had some very pleasant encounters with nurses, and a few unpleasant experiences. Once, I was in a hospital in St. Louis after a bad automobile accident. My skull was fractured and there was a suspicion of a broken back. I was more or less in a coma for a long time, and not allowed to move at all, which was fine as far as I was concerned, as I didn't want to move and didn't know whether I could if I tried. One morning, a doctor walked in and found a nurse changing my bed. She had me sitting up while she changed my pillows. I wasn't objecting because I wasn't conscious enough to talk or know what was happening. I later heard she was fired, which may have been drastic. But, leaving out the touchy condition of my head, no one, much less a nurse, moves a patient if there's even a suspicion that his back is broken.

Some weeks later, when my nurse was a nice, warm-hearted, middle-aged Irish woman and my progress had been steady, I ran into an unexpected roadblock. All of a sudden, something went wrong inside my battered head and my right side became paralyzed, from the neck up. This came on quite suddenly while I was eating lunch. I was having something that should have been innocuous, like soup, when I suddenly choked. Later, they realized that my semi-paralysis had set in at that moment and the muscles on one side of my throat stopped working, so the food wasn't being pushed down in the normal fashion. My nurse saw what was happening and that I was having trouble breathing. She tried sticking her finger down my throat to clear the problem by making me throw up, but nothing happened. So she opened the door, stepped out into the hall, and, finding a young intern going by, stopped him and said she needed help. He started to walk on, saying, "Sorry. This isn't my floor."

My nurse acted, instead of talking. She moved after the

intern, grabbed his arm, and pulled him into the room. She was probably twenty-five years older than he was, and twenty-five pounds heavier. "I've got a patient dying in here," she told him. "Now you stay here and do something!"

It worked. The two of them got me to throw up, cleared the obstruction, and I was able to breathe again. Soon the doctors were in, worrying about what had caused the sudden paralysis, and taping closed my right eye, as I had lost the power to close my eyelid and my eye was getting dry and hurting. There had obviously been an interruption in my nervous system, probably caused by internal (inside my head) bleeding. I found it difficult to eat for a time.

Until some muscles fail, you don't realize how much you use them for purposes you never think about. Until I had this minor misadventure, I hadn't realized how useful your cheek and tongue muscles are for eating; you need them badly to keep food in place so your teeth can chew it up, and then to move the chewed food around in your mouth so you can swallow it. This was a minor problem—I chewed everything on my left side until the paralysis went away. I recovered gradually, my improvement measurable by wrinkling my brow. When the paralysis was complete, only the left half of my forehead would wrinkle and the right side would stay clear. Eventually, my semiparalysis cleared up completely. I've always felt I was saved by the quick-wittedness and devotion to duty of a nurse. When I was able to think about it, I realized I had been appalled by the young doctor who tried to walk away because it wasn't his floor and so not his responsibility.

In hospitals, I have found that people usually receive the treatment they expect. I always expected to be treated well. I would say that, over all, I was treated better than most patients for a number of reasons. One is I'm a more experienced patient than most, and know what can and cannot be done in a hospital. I'm normally a cheerful person. I don't think I fall into the "cheerful cripple" category, but I was born with a sunny disposition and it shows. Like everyone else, I get blue or discouraged at times, but rarely for long. I'm not noisy, I rarely raise my voice, and while I can be stubborn, I don't ask for anything unreasonable and I don't make a fuss. In a comparatively short time, this is noticed and appreciated.

As a child, I was friendly and usually laughing. I suppose a pattern like that gets set and remains. I've always been surprised at how helpful people will be when you smile— when you smile and mean it, not when you grimace because you're trying to get something. I've been amazed that more people don't do it; it makes you feel better and has the same effect on others. I may have been influenced early by the theory that says we don't smile because we're happy, we're happy because we smile. And, conversely, we may cry because we're unhappy, but also we're unhappy because we cry. Whatever it is, I have been fortunate as a rule in my relationships with nurses and other staff members in hospitals.

A good, efficient nurse on a floor or in a department can make all the difference in the world to a patient. As shifts change, you can feel the mood of the patients change. Some perfectly good nurses are people who live by the book— everything must be done just so, at the appointed time. Others turn out to be just as good but more easy-going. Often, these types fool you—you can be taken in at first by a good-natured, take-it-easy nurse, only to discover that she isn't as nice as she seems, and that everything works better when the unsmiling, hard-driving nurse is on duty. I was fooled once by a hard-faced type who came on too strong at our first meeting, but realized after a few days that she was as good a nurse as I've ever seen. The whole floor operated better when she was on duty, and she had charge of only one segment of it.

Nurses, nurses' aids, and orderlies are around all the time; they are the people the patient has the most contact with, whereas the doctors are in evidence only occasionally. The situation can be compared to that of an airline and its passengers. The best pilots and maintenance service make flying safe and comfortable, but an airline's reputation with the flying public depends more on the stewardesses and ticket-counter help. These are the people the public sees most. In a similar way, much of a hospital's reputation with patients depends on the nurses and their helpers. Not only on how thoughtful, considerate, and efficient they are, but on how they get along with one another.

There was a time when registered nurses were usually white, and older. There were gradations in the scale, which the knowledgeable could determine by uniform, with the type of cap often the tip-off. Generally, the lower and more menial jobs were done by younger people working their way up, or by nonwhites or foreigners. Various forms of integration have had their effect, and, on the whole (from the patients' point of view), this has meant an improvement. A couple of years ago, I was a patient in a large, old hospital. The buildings certainly wouldn't have attracted anyone. But it was one of the nicest hospitals I was ever in, because the staff, particularly in the lower echelons, all got along well. Whites and blacks, Catholics and Protestants, natives and foreign-born, Puerto Ricans, Cubans, and other Latins all worked with each other according to their skills and training, with a maximum of good humor and cooperation and a minimum of clannishness. As there used to be such a thing at sea as a "happy ship," this was a happy hospital. Its physical set-up was outdated, but it had something more important which, for want of a better word, has to be called morale.

As a patient, it's usually easy to get along in a hospital. If an individual is thoughtful and considerate of others, he will usually be treated with consideration. There will always be cranky and selfish patients. Normally, they are not treated as well as the others, but usually they are treated better than they deserve to be. Hospital staffs often make allowances for them, falsely figuring that they may be pleasant people when well. In my experience, this is not true. People who are nice act nice when they're sick; people who aren't nice act worse —their less noble characteristics are accentuated.

A patient should learn the local ground rules and live up to them. So should his family and regular visitors and other guests. In any hospital with limited visiting, the patients' worst days, or nights, come after they've had visitors. There are many reasons for this, most of them obvious. There is an old saying about the wheel that creaks the loudest being the first to be greased. This doesn't work out well in most hospitals. The chronic complainer soon gets the worst service and treatment; the quiet one who doesn't ask for much will usually be treated much better. What one does as a patient depends on the regulations and customs of each hospital.

I have found it rarely hurts to keep a bottle of liquor around to offer to the staff when they're going off duty and can take a drink. Candy and cookies offered regularly cheer up cleaning women as well as doctors and nurses. Patients often get flowers, and it doesn't hurt any to offer them to the staff. A young intern or resident can take them along for his date, and a nurse, whether or not she has a date, is rarely insulted by an offer of flowers.

But those are physical things. The most important factor in

how a patient gets treated is his own attitude. What he gets back is really a reflection of what he gives out.

The entire attitude toward patients has changed in recent years. When I was young, sick children who could afford it recuperated in private rooms with private nurses. Now they're usually put into multibed rooms, for a very simple reason: they get well faster that way. This is also true of most adults. People who are ill may prefer privacy, but they can become too absorbed in themselves and their problems. They are usually better if they have to see other people and are made to realize that others also have problems and suffer. Post-operative treatment used to be based on making it a slow and gradual business. The theory was that the patient had had quite a shock to his nervous system, so he should be allowed time to get his strength back. Now the theory is: get them up and moving as soon as possible.

With the current nursing shortage and higher costs, more people are on general nursing care, and doing well on it. There are no hard and fast rules, of course, as everyone's illness is different, and so is every patient's personality. Some illnesses require different treatment; some people respond to one form of care, others to another. A hospital is like a school in a way—it can only do a certain amount with the raw material it gets. The one cannot make a moron brilliant, the other cannot make a malingerer well. Or make a chronic complainer into a happy, improving patient. The main impetus, as always, has to come from the individual.

CHAPTER ELEVEN

Motivation
and
Rehabilitation

Ever since I started thinking about this book, I have found I was spending more and more time on one aspect: motivation. There are really three key ideas: motivation, the individual, and rehabilitation. Why is one person knocked out by an apparently light blow while another gets hit by a haymaker and gets up repeatedly to keep fighting?

It is not popular or relevant today to talk about determination or willpower. According to some, there is no such thing —we are all products of so many forces we barely understand, the idea that we can determine our own destinies is preposterous.

Then what is it that makes the difference? Why do some people give up at the slightest adversity, while others fight against it for a time and then surrender, and some of the remainder fight against it as long as they live?

We've all seen examples. There doesn't seem to be any pattern to give a clue. After the end of World War II, when I was working for the State Department, I read a good many reports of relief agencies. I went over a number of studies of Greece, for instance, looking for a pattern. Greece had been invaded by the Nazis and then bedeviled by internal factional fighting. Much deprivation and starvation took place among the populace for years. Maybe one person in a family would seem unaffected physically, maybe three or four in a small village, and there was no explanation for it. Of several children, one might seem full of hope and determination while his brothers were lethargic. The more fortunate one was not always the oldest, always the youngest, or always the one in the middle. I was not able to find any common denominator.

There are certain people, of course, who are born survivors. Not always the nicest people, some of them survive catastrophes by being extremely self-centered and using others. Some seem to have survived various ordeals relatively untouched, in the same way some of the physically handicapped seem to have come through with their psyches intact. Not completely, of course. Everyone has to be affected by things that happen to him, but some turn out to be strong enough not to be destroyed by them. A psychiatrist would tell you that it isn't a matter of putting these unpleasant things behind you, because you can't bury disagreeable or unpleasant experiences; the best thing you can do is face them, realize that they happened. And then see what you can do to overcome or mitigate their effects.

I have operated on the theory that you can do what you want to do within reason, physical handicaps notwithstanding, if you want to do it badly enough to work at it. I don't think I would ever become a great or passable painter, no matter how I worked at it, but that wouldn't be because a physical handicap was preventing me, rather a mental or artistic one. Most of the things I felt were important for me to do, I have worked out a way to do. One of my failures was dancing. I say I did not consider that important enough to try to work out a way. Or was I afraid to risk it? Did I really not think it that important, or did I decide it wasn't necessary because I was afraid I wouldn't be able to do it? By this time, it makes very little difference. On the other hand, I considered golf important enough to give it some thought and work at it, and now I don't play at all. I believe it was important for me to be able to drive a car. But did I have to learn how to fly, or was that something I did for my ego?

The examples of people with physical handicaps who wanted to do something desperately enough to do it are so numerous that a long, dull list could be made of them. Some were undoubtedly compensating or overcompensating for their handicaps, others were just determinedly going along on a predetermined course, undaunted. Some of these seem to have gone to great pains to continue an activity from which they had apparently been excluded.

Douglas Bader of England is an example of this. A pilot, he lost both legs before World War II, and applied to reenter the R.A.F. when the war began. He was persistent and experienced, and the need was great. He kept at it until he talked the authorities into letting him rejoin the service as a fighter pilot. He became a group captain and an ace. Deprived of an opportunity to use his skill, he worked his way back to putting it to good use for his country.

In a different way, Franklin Delano Roosevelt did the same thing. FDR was a government figure—a state senator in 1910, Assistant Secretary of the Navy from 1913 through World War I, unsuccessful Vice-Presidential candidate, run-

ning with James Cox, in 1920, a year before he came down
with polio. His career, like Bader's, was interrupted by a
handicap but not stopped, and he got back on the path he
had chosen.

A man with a handicap such as Glenn Cunningham, the old
mile runner, is a different kind of case. Cunningham was
caught in a fire as an infant and was so badly burned it was
thought that he'd never be able to walk again. He not only
walked, but by the time he was in his twenties he was the
leading mile runner in the world, because he had the drive
and determination to overcome what could have been a crippling misfortune. Michael Flanders, the British satirist, per-
forms brilliantly on stage in a wheelchair. Herbert Marshall,
the actor, had a long and outstanding career that ignored the
fact that one of his legs was an artificial one.

As a writer and editor, I have never found that walking
with crutches was a major factor in what I was able to do. A
lack of mobility limited some of my activities, but this was
never serious. I always said that as a free-lance writer it gave
me a certain productive advantage. Almost any writer will
tell you that—except for certain moments when everything
is going smoothly—anything is better than writing. Therefore, when sitting down to work, he can think of dozens of
things that have to be done before he can settle down to
writing. Because I'm essentially lazy and getting up and moving about is an effort, once I sit down to the typewriter I'm
apt to stay there, ignoring the blandishments of fixing the
leaky faucet or going out to buy that reference book I'd like
but don't need. I can only blame my failures on myself, not
on the fact that I had polio a long time ago.

This whole matter of working, of being a useful member
of society, is a most important factor in the well-being and
self-esteem of the physically handicapped. That and success-

ful relationships with those of the opposite sex are the two vital factors in the total success of a handicapped person. Often, the two go together. A man who feels he can't work and contribute his share to society because of a physical handicap is not apt to attempt or be able to establish a real relationship with a woman. A woman with a handicap is apt to feel the same way. For many of the handicapped, rehabilitation begins with vocational rehabilitation.

There are a number of organizations working to help the handicapped in this way. They have different names and methods, but all seem to have one thing in common—they seem to be run by people who are more interested in doing something for others than in making money for themselves. Some of these organizations are run or managed by people who have handicaps, others are run by the hale. In either case, they should put to shame those people who make fun of so-called do-gooders. Most of these people could be put into that category and are at least as dedicated and hardworking as the most strenuous proponent of the profit motive.

One of the most interesting of these organizations is called Abilities, Inc., a firm on Long Island. It was started by Henry Viscardi, Jr., who was born with small twisted stumps for legs and didn't walk until he was twenty-six years old, when he was fitted with prostheses after surgery. Hank Viscardi started teaching other handicapped people how to walk and, in time, how to live.

Working on the assumption that the most important thing for the handicapped was employment, he started by trying to find jobs for them. He ran into so much prejudice in hiring practices that he established his own company, employing only the handicapped. Abilities, Inc., is not a manufacturer, but acts as a contractor for manufacturers, or for any other business to which Hank Viscardi and other salesmen can sell the skills of the five hundred disabled workers of Abilities, Inc. They work on light assemblies for manufacturers, they make up payrolls for other companies, they handle taxes and accounting for others. They do any number of jobs for many companies.

But the important thing is that they do these things at regular rates, competing in the open market, making their own livings by using skills they have developed. Working as an outside company, as a subcontractor at times, Abilities, Inc., often does work for companies that wouldn't hire handicapped employees in their own plants. Its first job used five men, lacing cable assemblies. The five had, between them, one good leg and seven good arms. But they had desire and spirit and five sound heads. From that small beginning, the firm has grown. And it has enabled hundreds of handicapped men and women to become self-supporting, to get, or get back, their self-respect.

Hank Viscardi and Abilities, Inc., have become an important feature in many lives. Viscardi also started and heads The Human Resources Foundation, which is the research division of Abilities, Inc.; he is a director of JOB (Just One Break) and is involved in other work to help those who need help.

There are a number of organizations and firms now trying to do something for the handicapped, most of them started by the efforts of one person to help others. JOB, for instance, is an employment agency, or placement agency, for the handicapped. It was started in 1949 by Orin Lehman, of the New York banking family, who had returned from World War II minus a leg. Lehman used his personality and connections to get a number of industrialists and financial people interested in the problem of jobs for the handicapped, and thus bring it before the public.

Various firms got involved in this type of work, for one reason or another. The Bulova watch people, for instance, run the Joseph Bulova School of Watchmaking, set up for the purpose of training the handicapped. The Renault automobile people in France have quite a program for training and employing the handicapped. All over the country there are services available to help the handicapped become able to help themselves. Some are fine and effective, some look and sound good but aren't very useful. The difference between the useful ones and those that put up a good front but don't deliver is usually in the energy and character of the moving spirit of the organization.

The government, federal, state, and local, backs certain programs for the handicapped and can furnish much information about where to find facilities that will be helpful. The Department of Health, Education, and Welfare, through its Social and Rehabilitation Service, Washington, D.C. 20201, will mail general and specific information on request. The Veterans Administration does much fine work in the rehabilitation field, with hospitals and training centers all over the country. It is, however, somewhat limited, as it can work only with people who have served in the armed forces. The various government agencies have one problem in common: what they are able to do in any field varies from year to year depending on the budget for that fiscal year.

With all the fine rehabilitation work being carried on, wherever you look, wherever you go in this field, you will find people trained by and referring to Dr. Howard Rusk. He has been a most successful innovator in rehabilitative practices, and, as such, has been honored by organizations and governments all over the world. He is a professor and chairman of the Department of Rehabilitation Medicine at the New York University Medical Center, where he heads the Institute of Rehabilitation Medicine. Most New Yorkers, and most people, don't know it by that name—it is almost universally known as the Rusk Institute.

One of the major aspects of rehabilitation today is in the field of prosthesis, which is the replacement of a limb or other part of the body with an artificial device. The change in the art of prosthesis since the end of World War II has been so pronounced that people accustomed to its earlier state are living in a different and outmoded world. The concept has changed from a make-do policy to an attempt to duplicate the work done by the missing or damaged parts. Progress has been rapid because of major improvements in biomedical technology and knowledge of the human body and how it works. Progress would be faster if parts whose functions have to be duplicated weren't so versatile. Very few portions of the human anatomy have a simple, single function the way teeth do.

The most common mechanical substitutes are for all or portions of the arms and legs. Unfortunately, limbs are among mankind's most complicated external parts. Only primates have the subtle and sophisticated joints that enable limbs to move in many directions, as well as many-fingered hands with opposed thumbs. They make man agile, dangerous, mobile, and tool-wielding. They also make life more difficult for the prosthesis maker.

For centuries, if a human lost or was born without a hand or arm or foot or leg, he got along without, or used a crude, usually wooden substitute. Around the turn of the century, with a mechanical age coming in, some complicated artificial limbs were produced with clumsy and cumbersome joints for articulation. But the great leap forward didn't take place until after World War II. It seems confusing and contradictory, but warfare, man's cruelest and most useless practice, often brings about the speediest and most spectacular progress in the field of healing.

For some time, medical people have been experimenting with different forms of homografts—putting back the severed leg of a dog, for instance, or replacing one dog's severed leg with the leg of another. The surgeons and physiologists learned a good deal about what could and could not be done, and in recent years have had some success with human homografts. Mainly, these orthopedic attempts were successful only when a dismembered portion of the body could be put back immediately in such a way that it might have a chance to grow back together and be functional again, in whole or in part. Internally, operations such as heart or kidney transplants were accomplishing the same things. But the replacement of a living member with a living member is not the same as replacing a living member with an artificial or mechanical member. A few of the problems are similar; most are completely different.

Transplant or any form of graft has to face the problem of compatibility, so that the body does not reject the new material. This is a problem long familiar to medical men but comparatively new to the world at large. As members of the lay public, we have listened and watched with awe and wonder and have learned a little about the matching of tissues and the delicate job of piecing together veins and arteries and muscles and nerves so that in time separate pieces can become functionally one again.

The first prosthetic devices of which most of us may have been aware were probably wooden arms, or legs, or artificial feet. We all got to know Captain Hook of *Peter Pan*, or Stevenson's Long John Silver, or perhaps, if we lived in the days of vaudeville, a dancer like Peg-Leg Bates. The point about Bates was that he had worked out an interesting and entertaining dance routine, not in spite of having one wooden leg but capitalizing on it.

For centuries, wooden and metal objects had been painstakingly fashioned into inert duplicates of missing parts and then fastened onto the body by various ingenious methods. As Samuel Johnson remarked when comparing women preachers with dogs walking on their hind legs, it is not done well, but you are surprised to find it done at all. That was a reasonable description of the results that could be achieved by hard-working, clever people using some of the early prostheses.

The great change began with the use of different materials. It is not easy to find something as light and strong as wood, as capable of being formed into shapes, as long-lasting and inherently resistant to variations in temperature, moisture, and other conditions. Modern plastics opened up a new world to makers and users of artificial limbs. This was followed by portable, longer-lasting power supplies, along with breakthroughs and developments in electronics and miniaturization.

The problems seemed endless. The different motions required by human joints such as the shoulder, elbow, wrist, hip, knee, and ankle—and we're not even mentioning fingers and toes—are not required by any nonprimate animal. Consider for a moment the different kinds of motion needed by the elbow, a truly universal joint that not only bends and straightens out but also rotates while bent or straight. Consider what the human leg does when climbing stairs or a ladder or a hill. Then try building something that can imitate all of these motions, something that can be *directed* to copy all of these functions, to perform in a like fashion.

The functions necessary for any specific prosthesis depend, of course, on what natural part it is replacing. Though it wouldn't seem to be the case, the functions of a prosthesis depend in part on whether one or both limbs have been affected. If one leg is missing, for instance, an artificial leg can be helpful if it does no more than support the body while the "good" leg is brought into place to make more delicate movements. If both legs have been lost, the replacements must be more sophisticated. The same thing holds true of arms and hands. Generally, when working, one hand is used as a "holder," the other as a tool or mover.

Barrie's Captain Hook was mentioned—a shaped piece of wood with a hook at the end was an early prosthesis and, in most ways, an effective one. It also had many drawbacks, as did all the older substitutes. And even the newest and most advanced ones are not true substitutes for missing parts; the best of them are devices that can simulate some human movements. That is not meant to sound defeatist or discouraging—the progress of the past ten years should prevent that.

One of the difficulties we mentioned is that a living part has a variety of movements. The capacity for many of these can be built into the substitute member, but this takes care of only one portion of the problem and ignores the need to control these movements. Progress in this has been both fast and slow. Captain Hook's primitive hook was just that, a hook. Today's version is called a split hook, a two-part device consisting of two hooks, at least one of which is movable and under control. This provides an artificial version of the opposed thumb and thus enables the wearer to grasp objects. This is a large step toward using tools, whether the tool is a pencil or an automobile steering wheel or the controls of a drill press.

The earlier movable prostheses were controlled mechanically—that is, by using some other muscle or muscles to actuate the artificial limb so it could be bent or straightened. The range of movement was limited and so was the control, and the prosthesis was hardly capable of delicate movements.

But it was better than nothing. To learn how to use one with even a modicum of success took a great deal of patience and ingenuity. As the new lightweight materials revolutionized the prosthetics industry, so have electronics and amplification systems. Miniaturization was needed, or the motor and power units would be too large and heavy to be portable. Whether the future is going to lie with such devices or with homografts is still a moot point.

At one time, and not so long ago, if one lost an arm or a hand or a finger, that was that. The attempts to replace them where they had been were clumsy efforts, although, whether or not they worked properly, they at least presented a better appearance by having something where there had been a noticeable lack. In recent years, with greater knowledge of antisepsis and the nature of tissue, it has proven possible to do more than sew back severed members, which was the first step. The procedure has advanced, step by step. It has long been known that bones could be placed so they would grow together and mend themselves, and under proper conditions, flesh will do the same. Modern techniques also reassemble muscles, tendons, and blood vessels. Now, in more spectacular fashion, nerve systems are put together so they can be reconnected or grow together and function normally.

In time, after more is known about compatibility and rejection, there will probably be spare-parts banks, like the eye banks, so that badly diseased or missing members can be replaced, with the replacements attached to functioning torsos and eventually functioning normally themselves. Until that time, we will have to make necessary repairs by using prostheses.

Some of the difficulties have been mentioned—mainly, the incredibly complicated processes that go into even the simplest activities. One can think of an animal's nervous system as being akin to the wiring of a computer. Only instead of a read-out, there is action. The impulses that pass through a nerve system are electric in nature and measurable. For most activities, the brain is the programmer of a computer system. Hundreds of thousands of times a day, the brain "programs" all our physical activities except those that are repeated so often in the same form they seem to be reflex actions.

If one wants to perform a simple action, such as picking up a glass of water, the brain sends out a regular torrent of instructions. It tells different muscles to get moving in a specific order so that the arm and hand extend to the glass, so that fingers curl around the glass, gently, not hard enough to crush it but hard enough so that it won't be dropped. And while it is so held, other muscles have to raise the glass, taking care to keep it level so the water doesn't spill. Perhaps, at the same time, the brain is sending out signals to the mouth and tongue, and perhaps to the legs and other parts of the body so the held glass can be carried to another person or to a different part of the room.

Carrying on such a simple activity with a prosthetic device is a task of such multiple complications that the physical aspects seem staggering. Using any form of split-hook device for grasping delicate objects requires a form of feedback mechanism so that the user, with no sense of feeling in the business end of the device, does not grasp so hard that the object is crushed. But the grasp must be firm enough so that the object doesn't slip. When prostheses were moved mechanically, this sensitivity was just about impossible; the means of measuring and controlling the use of the artificial muscles was too clumsy and coarse, without enough gradations.

The more modern forms of articulated limbs are moved by electricity, the stimulus is an electrical impulse, and the motive power comes from tiny electric motors. Pressure sensors in the "fingertips" feed back information on the amount of pressure being applied. These sensors are often connected with a form of locking device so that a predetermined amount of pressure can be applied without the impulse being steadily repeated, so a fragile thing may be held firmly but not crushed. It just happens that the normal control system for nerves and muscles works on a direct (for all practical purposes) linear system, which means that the strength of the muscular response varies directly with the strength of the stimulus, in this instance an electric current. Fortunately, that is the way electric motors react.

The locking device mentioned above works as a no-slip mechanism similar to locking pliers that can be set at one point and will remain at that point until released. This is handy in prosthesis, as it means no more current has to be used, once it is set, which is important when the user has to carry with him his electric supply system.

Many split-hook users have become amazingly deft in the manipulation of their devices both for delicate work and for power uses—handling tweezers, for instance, or a hammer. The earlier forms, actuated mechanically, were controlled by movements of the head or thumb or shoulder, almost anything that the user could control and that could be attached to the device. In recent years, attempts have been made to activate the device by using the same nerve signals that formerly activated the muscles. Usually, the nerves continue to the point of amputation, as we noted when discussing phantom pain. Much experimental work has been done along the lines of having the brain use the human nervous system until it can be connected with the controls of the prosthesis. This is still crude, but looks promising, and in time will probably be worked out, which will be a major step forward in the field.

While pressure sensors on the surface of the device allow for a sensitivity previous contraptions did not have, there are still many things that the best of prostheses cannot do or feel. Heat or pain, for instance, though these could be programmed into the device if such additional activity served a purpose useful enough to make it worth the extra trouble. The newer, more sensitive devices might stop one thing that drives prosthesis makers up the wall: the wearer's habit of using the device as a hammer or club. After all, it is handy (attached), it can't feel, isn't likely to be damaged, and can be controlled more directly than almost any other tool.

If any of this sounds as though the new prostheses have solved all the problems, that is not the case at all. No matter how good they are and how much they are improved, they remain substitutes. And they are not easy to operate; the proper way to use them has to be learned, which takes time, effort, and concentration. This is a real drawback, because often something that nature did without thinking about it can be done only with extreme concentration. Which means learning or relearning how to do simple things that were never before considered as tasks.

I have had to learn how to walk several times. The first time was as an infant, as most people do. After that, a few times as my physical condition and capacity changed drastically. I have never had to have prostheses, but a few of my experiences came close.

At one time, the only way I could stand up and walk (with crutches) was by wearing special metal braces that locked at the knee. I worked out my own system to make things simpler for me. Metal sleeves or rings fitted the two ends of the braces at the knee, where it bent. The sleeve, in its down position, kept the brace stiff for walking, as there wasn't enough muscle in my legs to support the weight of my body. In order for me to sit down, each sleeve, one on the inside, one outside, had to be lifted so the leg could bend. Reaching down and moving each by hand took time and trouble. I worked out a system whereby they were connected to a string or wire that went up inside my pants to my belt. A small upward hitch on the belt unlocked the brace. I'm over-simplifying this a bit, because one leg had a lock at the hip, too. The braces were made of steel, painted black, and leather. At points of use, where the sleeves fitted and were often moved, the paint wore off, and in a short time the metal would get rusty, and then my system, using a gentle hitch to unlock and gravity to lock, wouldn't work. In due time, the braces developed a certain smell of oil. Graphite lasted longer and was odorless, but got my clothes and hands dirty.

One of the purposes of prostheses is to enable the wearer to function, or function better than without it. Another is to remove the stigma or handicap or disadvantage of being different. A person with one limb may be able to function in many ways without serious loss of ability but he will always look different when so doing. As an extreme example, take the case of a singer. A one-armed piano player would have problems of a specific type, but a one-armed singer's main problem when performing would be one of appearance. Anyone can understand that a one-armed singer would feel better appearing on the concert stage, or anywhere else, with an artificial arm than with an empty sleeve, even though the vocal attempt might be the same. While many people want to be different from others, they want to be different in a way they consider positive—to be prettier or nicer or smarter. Few, if any, want to be different in a way that is immediately noticeable physically and that might re-pel some people.

A very important prosthesis factor, then, at least to the user, is its cosmetic function. For instance, the most efficient current artificial hand uses the split-hook type of device. Many users also have an artificial hand they can wear in its place, a hand that works much less efficiently but has no hooks, only four fingers and a thumb, even if they don't do any work. When appearing in public, a user may wear this hand—and take it off and put on the more practicable split hook when he gets home.

Not all the improvements in the field have been in the mechanical aspects. Improvements in the cosmetic aspects of artificial limbs have been at least as pronounced and just as important to the user. Modern science and technology, which have made so many original products, have come up with a synthetic covering that isn't skin but does everything except perspire when nervous and could do that if necessary. A form of it is used on the split hook described earlier, so it can carry and hold in a nonskid grip the glass mentioned before, or a hammer, or a piece of candy. The plastic skin can be put on an artificial finger or hand, and be matched with the skin of the user, even to imitating his fingerprints.

Prosthetic devices used to be held on by straps, sleeves, or collars that were bulky and unsightly. Today, they are apt to be attached by what are, in effect, suction cups. These take some getting used to, but so did the straps, and the new method is generally more efficient and looks so much better that it is often difficult to tell where nature leaves off and artifice begins.

Advances in prostheses are going on apace. People are able to wear them now in more comfort than before, and to perform in them in a way that wasn't conceivable a few years ago. There is no reason to think that the rate of these improvements will be slowed. The main question is the direction the future will take. Will it make more human the abilities and appearance of these artificial devices or will it move eventually in the direction of human grafts? The parts do not have to come from our own bodies. What is the difference between living with another person's kidney or heart inside you and walking on what had been another person's leg? And if either or all of them work, is the difference important?

Of course, with the heart transplants we have run into an ethical problem. Death has had to be reconsidered. If death takes place when the heart stops beating, which heart—the original or the transplanted one? Or when blood to the brain has been stopped long enough for the brain to stop functioning, what are we going to do when we move to the kind of operation described in science fiction, where we substitute parts of the brain or even the whole brain? Then we run into the problem of who is doing what. Is the brain that commanded the arm to pick up the rifle, aim it, and shoot it responsible for murder, or is it the artificial finger or hand that pulled the trigger? Legally, thinking of a crime, only thinking of it, is not a crime. The crime is in carrying it out.

In the spring of 1972, a patent was issued to a man who had lost his right hand in 1958 playing with firecrackers. The patent was for something he had devised, an artificial hand with an adapter to hold a violin bow so that the bow can pivot when being played. The inventor is an engineering technician who taught himself to play the violin using an artificial hand. It didn't work quite right, so he invented a bow holder that rests in the palm and pivots as needed. This is a man who wanted to do something—play the violin—and couldn't do it properly because he'd lost a hand in a childhood accident. But he wanted to make music his way and wanted it with enough intensity so that he worked out a way to do it, and now others with the same problem will be able to play.

With prostheses, as with anything used by the handicapped, the device is not as important as the will to use it, the desire to make it work, the push to make an imperfect body perform. The thing that makes life worth living for the handicapped is hope and desire and work toward leading a normal life, toward being a part of the mainstream of the society in which we live, being able to contribute something more to mankind than our small physical presence. With this, we come back to the major question of motivation.

There can be no general answer to the question of what motivates an individual. The physical problems are different in each case; every person varies in the way he will respond to his problems and to attempts by others to get him to cope with them. The doctors and therapists working with the handicapped differ in approaches and methods, according to their own temperaments and training.

I have spent a good deal of time talking to people who deal with these problems, and find no agreement, no set theories as to what will work. The ones new in the field are the most apt to come up with didactic answers. The more experienced successful practitioners say the methods change according to the patient and his needs. The most discouraging thing is to be unable to get any response, to find the patient going along dully, doing what is suggested or recommended but without any spark.

One fine doctor who gave up a good surgical practice to work with rehabilitation of the disabled told me about one of his patients. "He was about eighteen, a promising young athlete when he was injured in an auto accident. It was a spinal injury, and he lost all the use of one leg and much of the ability of the other. Like his parents, he was not a well-educated man. He, and they, could read and write, but took little interest in anything outside of their immediate lives or their household. So he had no resources on which to fall back. He stayed in his section of the hospital, content to be taken care of as well as the institution could. He showed little interest in anything—other patients, what was going on around him or in the world.

"It was difficult to get him to answer questions, and he never offered a word on his own. I watched him when he had visitors, who were few, and he was the same with them all. His parents came every Sunday, but it obviously was an ordeal for them and for him. He didn't complain, he didn't cause trouble, he didn't do anything. It is natural after a serious accident for a patient to go into a state of shock, but he had stayed in one. I tried to arouse some emotion in him, some sign of life. I tried to make him angry, but that didn't work too well either, so I did something a little dangerous. I got him to rail against fate or whatever it was that had caused his accident, that had done this to him.

"He couldn't get angry at anyone else—he had been driving alone when he had skidded against a curb and been pinned in the car for some time. I put together what had happened to him physically and his promise as an athlete, and it worked. It got a response, and I built on that. Raging at a fate that caused one's trouble is usually counter-productive, but in time I was able to turn it into something positive, an ambition to show whoever or whatever it was that had engineered this for him that he wasn't going to be stopped this way.

"Today, he still has no power in one leg and only a little in the other. But he is out of the hospital, living at home with his parents and no longer apathetic. He is working with his physical therapist to regain some control over the muscles in his 'good' leg, and keeps after me to see if there isn't some nerve operation that might help. There doesn't seem to be, but with the progress we're making in neurosurgery, who knows? He's still a young man, and anything, almost anything, is possible."

This doctor was echoing the words I've heard from so many rehabilitation people I've talked to, phrased in one way or another—"After seeing that, I'll never again say anything is impossible."

What is it that makes it possible for some people to do the seemingly impossible? We're back again to motivation. What motivates a person to keep going, to fight back? It has to start somewhere, with a modicum of self-respect, a feeling of worth.

The trouble is that while outsiders, trained or otherwise, sometimes can help, as did the doctor who aroused rage in his apathetic patient, the motivation has to come from within almost every time. It has to be felt by the person involved; it can rarely be given to him. It isn't as simple as just wanting to do something, it has to be a burning, passionate desire. The motivation that makes a person with a physical handicap do everything he can, and a little more, to overcome it or lessen its effects probably has the same base as that which causes some nonhandicapped people to stay alive despite odds, or to become successful doctors or playwrights or parents. But as this book is supposed to be about the physically handicapped, I kept trying to get answers from the people who worked with them, and the only consensus I could get was in no agreement.

I tried a successful, very nice psychiatrist who does not specialize in the physically handicapped. He stopped to think before answering. "I was trained as a Freudian," he said. "But when I think about your question, I may have to go back on some of the things I was taught and answer that I think it's in the genes. Some people are born with this form of determination, self-respect if you will, and some are not. And if they have it, nothing that happens to them will take it away. Similarly, few will gain it, no matter how fortunate their circumstances. You can blame it on, or credit it to, heredity, though when you look at some of their parents, you wonder. But you realize you may have to go back many generations to find the combination of dominant and recessive traits that showed up in the generation now alive."

I've always considered myself a person with many faults, one of which is being stubborn. The other side of that is that it never occurs to me to give up when things look black. When my psychiatrist friend was telling me it was in the genes, it reminded me of a flip remark I'd made to my mother. She broke her hip a few years ago, when she was in her upper eighties, and when I saw her a year later, she was getting around badly, able to walk only with a "walker." Six or eight months later, when I drove out to see her again, she was standing by the window of her living room, waiting to show me how she was walking—without the walker, without crutches, without even a cane. Not well, but she was walking.

"Aren't you proud of me?" she asked.

"I certainly am," I said. I was quite moved, but if I ever said anything sentimental to my mother, she would think she must be on her deathbed. "You must have inherited it from me," I added.

I had always thought that if I had inherited anything from my parents, I had gained a certain quickness of mind from my mother, and determination from my father. I suddenly realized I had possibly received some of my stubbornness or determination from both sides of the family.

CHAPTER TWELVE

Conclusions

Having undergone the experiences that come to anyone with a physical handicap, you will have had to develop a philosophy of some kind, whether or not you call it that, and you must have come to some conclusions.

The first thing you have to do if you're going to make any kind of life for yourself is face facts. You don't have to make them any worse than they are, just realize what they are. You have to see a spade as a spade, not euphemize it as a manual earth-mover nor play it up as a god-damned shovel. No matter what you call it or how you look at it, it's just a spade, no more, no less. And you are a person, heroic, uncomplaining, indomitable, or bravely hiding your shivering cowardice—but still a person, an individual. And that is a basic fact that cannot be forgotten. You're a person first, a cripple or a person with a handicap second.

One of the facts you have to face is that life is not going to be a bed of roses. It isn't for anyone, and it will be harder for you. You aren't completely like other people and never will be. There is no use in trying to pretend that you aren't set apart to a certain extent by your handicap. How much you are set apart depends on how you handle your handicap and yourself. You can become accustomed to it, you can be so accustomed to it that everyone around you forgets it or takes it for granted, as you do, but you can't get rid of it by pretending it doesn't exist.

There will be times of joy and pleasure and accomplishment, and times of discouragement, of aching loneliness, usually because others are engaged in some activities you're prevented from doing. And before you feel too sorry for yourself at these times, you should remember that such depressions also come to other people—not only to you because of your handicap, but to the able-bodied, too.

Life is going to be more expensive for you than for others, even without figuring in medical expenses. The same degree of comfort, the same amount of "fun" will probably cost you more than it will the able-bodied. If it is a matter of transportation, you may not be able to use public methods, which means getting from place to place will cost you more. If you're going to a ballgame, a theater, an opera, you may have to buy the most expensive seats so you won't have to climb too far. There will be some movie houses you won't be able to attend because they're too hard to get in and out of, particularly when crowded.

I've mentioned the physical difficulty of getting into most hospitals and medical buildings—the same thing is true of many public and commercial buildings. More and more of them are being built without easy, straight, direct access from the street; too often, there is a stairway or escalator that makes it difficult for anyone in a wheelchair or with a mobility problem.

If it is a matter of housing, you may not be able to get around or be comfortable or safe in many less-expensive houses or neighborhoods. Even shopping or marketing may require a store where you can order by phone or that will deliver, all of which usually costs more. Also, you may find it's either difficult or dangerous for you to be in crowds. Even clothing is apt to be more costly; in many cases, ready-made patterns will not do and clothing will have to be tailored to your physical idiosyncrasies.

The important thing is to learn to use what you have rather than bewail what you don't have. I have said repeatedly that I consider myself lucky. Not because I have a physical handicap—far from it, I don't recommend that for anyone. One of the reasons is that I have survived, that things weren't worse.

Another is that I have a sort of mechanical sense. This is not something that you can learn; you can learn that certain things can or can't be done, but either you're born with an intuitive mechanical sense or you're not. It has made it easier for me to walk with crutches, say, and do some physical things that would be more difficult or more dangerous if they had to be learned rather than understood automatically. You can learn about centers of gravity and vectors and angles of incidence and the like. But if you're born with this mechanical sense, you know these things and how to use them to your advantage without having to learn them and the theories behind them.

I've often been bothered watching handicapped people walk, watching them do things dangerous to them, things that made their lives more difficult. Take, for example, walking with crutches on a slippery surface. You know instinctively or you learn by experience to take very short steps in these circumstances. The closer to the perpendicular your crutches and feet are, the smaller is your chance of slipping. That is an overly simple example, but it has amazed me how many handicapped people haven't learned it, or had to learn it the hard way, without understanding the reasons.

You have to learn how to take advantage of what you have. I was surprised to hear a doctor and physical therapist express amazement because one of his patients, without the strength to lift her foot over a high curb, swung her leg loosely in a pendulumlike manner so she was able to get it to the top of the curb and continue. What surprised me was not that she was able to do it but that the doctor was amazed. I realized she was using a trick I had learned many years ago —when your muscles aren't strong enough to do what you want them to do, you can often find a way to use momentum or some other natural force to accomplish what you want. The principle of the switchback to ascend a steep slope works just as well for a person without the physical strength to climb a hill as it does for a car or truck without enough horsepower to climb straight to the top of a mountain.

Although the handicapped are set apart by the fact of their handicap, generally that is because that is the way others see them; fundamentally, they are the same as everyone else. No two people are alike; all are shaped by the things that have happened to them. People tend to think of the handicapped as being alike because what the outsiders notice first is the physical thing that sets them off from the others.

Friends, relatives, and other outsiders will try to help you, and sometimes they can with some external, unimportant things. But they can't feel your pain or protect you from it. In the long run, you have to do the important things yourself.

This has its compensations. While no one else can feel your

pain, you know your accomplishments are your own. When an obstacle has been surmounted, you are the one who has overcome it.

If you believe in yourself, if you work at it, you can do anything within reason. And you can keep setting your sights higher so that more and more things come within the range of reason.

You can do it.

Addendum

There is a statement early in this book that since the introduction and widespread use of the Salk and Sabin vaccines polio has practically disappeared in the United States. As of now, that statement is still true. But it could change at any moment.

There has not been a polio epidemic in this country for many years. But health authorities are worried by the public's blithe acceptance of the idea that polio is no longer a menace. They have figures to back up their concern.

In 1955, there were 13,808 reported cases of paralytic polio. By 1961, the number of cases reported had dropped to 829. Ten years later, in 1971, 19 cases were reported, most of them in one section of the country. None of these 19 cases had received immunization treatment.

The percentage of preschool-age children who received the proper immunizing treatment, over 90 percent in 1964, had dropped year by year until it was about 63 percent (62.9) in 1972. The year before it had been 67 percent.

Polio has always been a truly democratic disease, striking alike the impoverished and the affluent, hitting just as hard at homes in the fancy suburbs and on Park Avenue as in the slums. This, too, could change. While the national average showed 63 percent had been properly immunized, in the lower-income areas the figures were 43 percent.

Before the vaccines were introduced, in the mid-1950s, the feeling among doctors had been growing that more people, particularly children, had contracted polio than had been realized. If they had had a mild case and suffered no aftereffects, it was usually diagnosed improperly as a cold or some childhood ailment. Doctors were slowly raising the percentage of people who had had polio without realizing it, when the question became moot because the vaccines put the whole problem in a different light. The only test for polio was by means of a spinal tap, an uncomfortable procedure that could not be used on everyone just to prove a point, particularly when the point no longer seemed relevant. Anyone who had once had polio was immune thereafter, which may have been one of the reasons that polio seemed to come in epidemics as new groups of children reached the most susceptible age.

Now, however, a generation has grown up with no "natural" immunity, as the disease has not been prevalent. And one child out of three has not been immunized by the vaccines before entering school. The conditions for an epidemic are building. One could start at any time, with a resulting tragedy in the form of many crippled and dead children.

Even one child who dies now from polio, or grows up without the full use of his limbs, is a totally unnecessary sacrifice to sloppiness, carelessness, or overconfidence. The vaccines are free and available. Parents should make sure that their children are immunized. Their doctors, health clinics, hospitals, and public health facilities can see to it. It is a simple, free, and painless procedure. For the slightly older group, school administrators should make sure that *all* children have been immunized.

Allowing a disease that has been effectively eliminated to return is another form of murder.

Bibliography

Abt, L. E. *Psychological Adjustments of the Amputee*. New York: McGraw-Hill Book Company, 1954.

Ayrault, Evelyn West. *Helping the Handicapped Teenager Mature*. New York: Association Press, 1971.

Elliott, Ruth. *Life and Leisure for the Physically Handicapped*. London: Elek Books, Ltd., 1971.

Feinstein, Luce, and Langstrom. *Influence of Phantom Limbs*. New York: McGraw-Hill Book Company, 1954.

Garrett, James F., and Levine, Edna S., eds. *Psychological Practices with the Physically Disabled*. New York: Columbia University Press, 1962.

Hewitt, Sheila, and John and Elizabeth Newsom. *The Family and the Handicapped Child*. Chicago: Aldin-Atherton, Inc., 1970.

Kessler, Henry Howard. *Rehabilitation of the Physically Handicapped*. New York: Columbia University Press, 1953.

Landis, C., and Bolles, M. M. *Personality and Sexuality of the Physically Handicapped Woman*. New York: Harper & Brothers, 1942.

Rochlin, Gregory. *Griefs and Discontents: The Forces of Change*. Boston: Little, Brown and Company, 1965.

Rusk, Howard A. *Living with a Disability*. New York: Blakiston, 1953.

———. *A World to Care For*. New York: Random House, 1972.

Shaffer, Laurance F., and Shoben, Edward J., Jr. *The Psychology of Adjustment,* 2nd ed. Boston: Houghton Mifflin Company, 1956.

Von Hilsheimer, George. *Special Child: A Handbook for Behavior Change.* Washington, D.C.: Acropolis Books, 1970.

Viscardi, Henry, Jr. *Laughter in the Lonely Night.* New York: Paul S. Eriksson, Inc., 1961.

Index

Pain *(cont'd)*
for alleviating, 84–85; energy required for fighting, 84; and fainting, 86; and "mind over matter," 86, 90; after operation, 58; phantom, 76–77, 180; and radio as distraction, 84–85; and reading as distraction, 85; subjectivity of, 80, 91; types of, 81
Pan American World Airways, 121
Parking, special, 126; *see also* Special Vehicle Identification (SVI) cards
Pediatrics, 156
Phantom pain, 76–77, 180
Physicians, *see* Doctors
Pity, 64–78 *passim*
Plane travel, by handicapped, 117–121
Plastic prostheses, 176
Plastic skin, 183
Poker, game of, 41
Poliomyelitis, 1, 6, 11, 152, 195; aftereffects of, 4, 55; possibility of new epidemic of, 196; statistics on, 195; test for, with spinal tap, 196
Pool, game of, 41
Popularity, desire for, 62
Pride, among handicapped, 32–46 *passim*
Prostheses, 174, 175–184; amplification system for, 178; attachment of, 183; cosmetic function of, 182–183; electrically moved, 179–180; and electronics, 176, 178; mechanically moved, 177, 179, 180; and miniaturization, 176, 178; nervous system connected with controls of, 180; plastic, 176; wooden, 175, 177
Psychoanalysis, 160

Queenie (dog), 19

Railway travel, 116
Rehabilitation, 8, 110; and motivation, 167–174, 185–188; vocational, 171–174; *see also* Prostheses
Renault training and employment program, 173
Rental car, 113, 114, 116, 119; Avis, 121; Hertz, 121
Roosevelt, Franklin D., 152, 155, 169–170
Roosevelt, Sara, 152
Rusk, Howard, 173
Rusk Institute, 174

Sabin vaccine, 1, 195
Salk vaccine, 1, 195
Self-confidence, among handicapped, 34
Self-pity, 65, 66, 67, 68, 71, 72, 76, 77, 78
Sex life, of handicapped, 128–145 *passim*, 171
Sheridan, Mary, 92
Shoes, special, use of, 11, 13
Skin, plastic, 183
Social and Rehabilitation Service (HEW), 173
Special Vehicle Identification (SVI) cards, 122, 123, 124, 125, 126
Split hook, 177, 179, 180, 183
Stevenson, Robert Louis, 16, 42
Sunrise at Campobello, 152
Surgery, orthopedic, *see* Orthopedic operation
Sverdlik, Sam, ix
SVI (Special Vehicle Identification)